Contact Lenses

Contact Lenses

Ken Daniels, OD

Assistant Clinical Professor
Director of Contact Lens Research
Pennsylvania College of Optometry
Private Practice: Hopewell and Lambertville, NJ

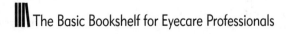 The Basic Bookshelf for Eyecare Professionals

Series Editors: Janice K. Ledford, COMT • Ken Daniels, OD • Robert Campbell, MD

SLACK
INCORPORATED
6900 Grove Road, Thorofare, NJ 08086

Publisher: John H. Bond
Editorial Director: Amy E. Drummond
Assistant Editor: Lauren E. Biddle

Daniels, Ken.
    Contact lenses / Ken Daniels.
        p. cm. -- (The basic bookshelf for eyecare professionals)
    Includes bibliographical references and index.
    ISBN 1-55642-345-4 (alk. paper)
    1. Contact lenses. I. Title. II. Series.
RE977.C6D36 1999
616.7'523--dc21   99-23383
                                                                                  CIP

Published by: SLACK Incorporated
                    6900 Grove Road
                    Thorofare, NJ 08086-9447 USA
                    Telephone: 609-848-1000, 856-848-1000
                    Fax: 609-853-5991, 856-853-5991
                    World Wide Web: http://www.slackinc.com

Contact SLACK Incorporated for more information about other books in this field or about the availability of our books from distributors outside the United States.

Authorization to photocopy items for internal or personal use, or the internal or personal use of specific clients, is granted by SLACK Incorporated, provided that the appropriate fee is paid directly to Copyright Clearance Center, 222 Rosewood Drive, Danvers, MA 01923 USA, 978-750-8400. Prior to photocopying items for educational classroom use, please contact the CCC at the address above. Please reference Account Number 9106324 for SLACK Incorporated's Professional Book Division.

For further information on CCC, check CCC Online at the following address: http://www.copyright.com.

Last digit is print number: 10 9 8 7 6 5 4 3 2 1

Dedication

This book is dedicated to the memory of loved ones past,
my mother and grandparents;
my family;
and most importantly,
to my beloved wife and best friend, my Judy.

Contents

Acknowledgments

Many thanks to SLACK Incorporated, John Bond, and Amy Drummond for asking me to be part of this endeavor. In particular, I salute and thank Jan Ledford for her perseverance and determination in helping me edit this book.

About the Author

Dr. Ken Daniels has been a clinical investigator for many of the manufacturers of contact lenses, medical devices, and ophthalmic pharmaceuticals. After graduating from the New England College of Optometry in 1987, Dr. Daniels joined Morrison Associates in Harrisburg, PA. He then joined Allergan–American Hydron Contact Lens Division in 1990 as the Manager of Clinical Development, and also spent time collaborating on research projects at the Cornea and Contact Lens Research Unit (CCLRU) at the University of New South Wales in Sydney, Australia. Dr. Daniels served as an Assistant Clinical Professor at the SUNY College of Optometry on his return from Australia. He is presently an Assistant Clinical Professor: Director of Contact Lens Research, and an NEI investigator for Collaborative Longitudinal Evaluation of Keratoconus (CLEK) at the Pennsylvania College of Optometry (PCO). He is also in private practice in Hopewell, NJ.

Dr. Daniels serves as the optometric editor of *The Basic Bookshelf for Eyecare Professionals*. He was a columnist for *Primary Care Optometry News* and presently serves as a consulting editor for *Optometry Today*.

Additionally, he serves the profession as the Educational Chair for Symposium 1999 and the Institutional Affairs Committee Chair for the American Optometric Association: Contact Lens Section. Dr. Daniels is a frequent lecturer at various optometric and ophthalmologic meetings on the topics of contact lens, refractive surgery, corneal topography, and anterior segment disease.

Introduction

From the early concepts of Leonardo Da Vinci (who wrote about "the human eye and methods of light entry into the eye through various materials" in 1508) to Descartes (who determined that water that comes into contact with the human eye neutralizes the power of the cornea in 1637) and Phillipe De La Hire (who described refraction of light at the anterior surface of the cornea and at the anterior and posterior surfaces of the lens in 1685), the idea of "corrective lenses" have come a long way.

The credit for the development of contact lenses and the understanding of optics belongs to many. Individuals such as Thomas Young, Eugene Fick (who described corneal irregularities that would be amenable to the placement of glass called a "Contactbrillen"), Jean Bapiste Kalt, Coques de Verre, August Muller, Carl Zeiss, Joseph Dallos, Theodore Obrig, George Nissel, Kevin Touhy, and Otto Witcherle were all engineers of the "art of fitting contact lenses." Authors such as I are simply the storytellers.

It is impossible in a few short pages to explain every nuance of contact lens fitting, an "art" that takes years of experience. It is my goal to assist in the learning process and enhance the experiential portion of education. This book touches only the surface of the field of contact lenses, but should provide a substantial foundation for furthering your knowledge.

What the Patient Needs to Know

- Contact lenses are an alternative to the visual correction of the eye.

- Contact lenses are medical devices which need to be properly maintained.

- A contact lens should always give good vision and good comfort, without redness or inflammation.

The Study Icons

The Basic Bookshelf for Eyecare Professionals is quality educational material designed for professionals in all branches of eyecare. Because so many of you want to expand your careers, we have made a special effort to include information needed for certification exams. When these study icons appear in the margin of a *Series* book, it is your cue that the material next to the icon (which may be a line, a paragraph, or an entire section) is listed as a criteria item for a certification examination. Please use this key to identify the appropriate icon:

OptA   optometric assistant

OptT   optometric technician

OphA   ophthalmic assistant

OphT   ophthalmic technician*

OphMT   ophthalmic medical technologist

LV   low vision subspecialty

Srg   ophthalmic surgical assisting subspecialty

CL   contact lens registry*

Optn   opticianry

RA   retinal angiographer

*Because these icons apply to the entire text, they will not appear anywhere on the pages.

Chapter 1

Contact Lenses and Ocular Anatomy

KEY POINTS

- Contact lenses will "fatigue" the tear production, decreasing the effects of the lacrimal system and increasing the potential for lens deposits, microbial infection, and corneal infiltration and edema.

- Dry eye tends to occur at a significant rate in 20% to 30% of contact lens patients.

- The average blink rate is approximately 7 blinks per minute, which increases to approximately 18 to 20 blinks per minute with the initial insertion of the contact lens.

- The tear film and epithelium act as barriers to foreign bodies and microorganisms as well as protection against friction during blinking.

- A peripheral zone, starting from the 4 to 5 mm mark out to the corneoscleral juncture, encircles the central corneal cap.

- The keratometer is designed to measure the center of the corneal cap, limiting the measurement to approximately 1.5 mm (approximately 8% of the corneal surface).

- Computer Assisted Corneal Topography (CACT) utilizes a video image capture system that allows for computer processing via a series of software applications.

- CACT is used to determine and document the shape and contours of the cornea. It is used to determine the amount and position of astigmatism.

Introduction

Contact lenses are medical devices supported by the lids, cornea, conjunctiva, and tear film. Contact lenses act as a physical barrier to normal tear-cornea-lid mechanics and corneal metabolism. This barrier effect can lead to various adverse reactions primarily related to oxygen deprivation. It is vastly important to understand normal anatomical and metabolic relations and how they are affected by the introduction of a contact lens to the eye.

Tear Film and Tear Function

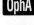

The tears can be adversely affected by the introduction of a contact lens to the ocular environment, leading to patient complaints of "dryness."

The volume of the tear fluid is approximately 7 microliters (±2), with 95% of the volume being produced by the lacrimal gland. Glands and cells of the lids and conjunctiva produce the rest of the components. Fifty percent of the tear volume is located along the lid margin and is called the tear meniscus or lacrimal lake. The rest is spread over the cornea and conjunctival surfaces by the lids. The tears have a normal pH level of 7.3 and a salt concentration of 0.91 to 0.97%. Normal tear evaporation is approximately 1 to 2 microliters per minute (15% of the total volume per minute).

The pre-corneal tear film has three layers: the oil layer, aqueous layer, and mucin layer. All three together are about 6 to 9 micrometers thick.

The first (outermost) layer of the precorneal tear film is the lipid layer, produced by the meibomian glands and the accessory sebaceous glands of Zeis (which are embedded in the superior and inferior lids). These glands secrete a partially solid oil and wax mixture. The gland openings are located on the lid margin anterior to the juncture of the conjunctiva and the epidermal layer of the lid. The lipids help stabilize the tear film and help prevent tear evaporation. If the spread of the lipid is insufficient, as is seen with surface elevations such as scars, pterygium, and pingueculae, the overlying surface will be susceptible to dryness due to tear evaporation and secondary exposure.

The optical quality of the eye is highly dependent on the integrity of the lipid layer. A depleted lipid layer will cause a disruption to the even spread of the tears and cause an irregularity in the precorneal surface. Such irregularities can cause power variations across the corneal surface, resulting in visual distortion.

The lacrimal gland and the accessory glands of Krause and Wolfring produce the aqueous (middle) layer. This layer is composed of a complex series of salts, sugars, urea, and proteins. Lactoferrin, an iron-carrying protein (similar to hemoglobin in the blood) supports oxygen transfer and demonstrates significant bacteria-inhibiting characteristics.[1, 2]

The mucus layer is the thinnest, innermost layer. It is produced by the conjunctival goblet cells, and creates an interface between the aqueous layer and the corneal epithelium. The corneal epithelial surface is hydrophobic ("water fearing"). The mucin layer reverses the hydrophobic characteristic of the epithelium to hydrophilic ("water loving"). Mucin also reduces the friction between the palpebral conjunctiva and the corneal epithelium during the blink.

The spread of the tear film over the cornea/contact lens system is critical to the success of contact lens wear. The eyelids spread the tear film like a windshield wiper on the car. The motion of the upper lid sweeps the tears downward and medially while the lower lid sweeps the tears upward and medially. This motion spreads the tear film evenly over the cornea surface and forces it towards the puncta for drainage into the canaliculi.

Blinking and spreading of the tear film is dramatically interrupted by the presence of a contact lens. The average blink rate is approximately 7 blinks per minute. This increases to approximately 18 to 20 blinks per minute with the initial insertion of the contact. Based on the comfort level of the patient and the contact lens material, the rate change may be even more dramatic. The effect is directly proportional to the material, such that polymethylmethacrylate (PMMA) (hard) > rigid (silicone acrylate [SA] > fluorinated silicone acrylate [FSA]) > hydrophilic (truncated > spherical). When the blink is altered, the blink rate becomes erratic and incomplete. This leads to a decrease in the proper spread of the tear film. This will cause subsequent lens dehydration and ocular discomfort.

A contact lens also acts as a barrier to sensation, contributing to an incomplete blink. Essentially, the lid does not know whether or not it has completely closed due to the lack of feedback. Incomplete lid closure leads to superficial corneal and conjunctival staining. This may trigger the release of biochemicals that cause conjunctival swelling (chemosis), redness (injection), and discomfort.

Corneal Anatomy and Contact Lenses

The cornea is comprised of the following layers: epithelium, Bowman's layer, stroma, Descemet's membrane, and endothelium. The cornea is the most powerful refracting surface of the eye, with an average diopteric power of 48.8.

The epithelium is 5 to 6 cell layers thick. The epithelium is the anterior continuation of the conjunctival epithelium (which is actually a continuation of the epidermis of the skin). The epithelium is anchored to the second layer of the corneal, the stroma, by a basement membrane called Bowman's membrane or layer. The epithelium has an average thickness of 50 to 60 microns.

The optical quality of the cornea depends on the integrity of the epithelium. The optical properties can easily be disturbed due to fluid changes or trauma induced by contact lenses. The tear film and epithelium act as a barrier to foreign bodies and friction (from blinking). With contact lens use, the corneal epithelium may have a loss of structural integrity leading to a greater sensitivity of the underlying nerve endings. Disturbance to epithelial function can be directly linked to a contact lens that reduces the available oxygen to the cornea. This situation is referred to as induced corneal hypoxia (see Chapter 10). Associated with this is an increase in carbon dioxide (hypercapnia).

The stromal layer is immediately posterior to Bowman's layer. The final, inner layer is the corneal endothelium, which is a single-celled layer 5 microns thick. The endothelial cells, which cannot regenerate, average 18 micrometers wide and are tightly joined. The endothelium keeps the corneal layers dehydrated. (The corneal epithelial surface needs to be hydrated by the tears, but the interior must be dehydrated in order to remain clear. A hydrated cornea becomes opaque.)

When the cornea is stressed, as during contact lens wear, the fluid balance shifts and the endothelial pump mechanism is unable to maintain the proper hydration of the cornea. This imbalance will lead to stromal edema. Edema is evidenced as either striae (moderate edema) or folds (severe edema).

Corneal hypoxia is the outcome of oxygen deprivation or depletion to the cornea associated with contact lenses. When the eye is open, the cornea acquires its oxygen supply from the atmosphere, aqueous, and limbal blood vessels. With the introduction of the contact lens to the eye, the oxygen supply is shifted to depend more on the oxygen supply from the aqueous humor. The shift is further extenuated when the eye is closed (eliminating atmospheric oxygen) and additional oxygen must be supplied by blood vessels. This creates a lower oxygen tension, leading to a shift in the fluid influx into the corneal stroma.

Hypoxia is directly proportional to the wear time. Long-term contact lens use (extended > flexible > daily, and soft > rigid) will have various hypoxic effects on the cornea. The amount of hypoxia and subsequent edema will be directly proportional to the length of lens wear.

OptA

The limbus, which forms the juncture between the cornea and the sclera, can also suffer from hypoxia. It may demonstrate new blood vessel growth called neovascularization. Normal limbal vascularization is differentiated from neovascularization by the physical characteristics of the vessels. Normal limbal vessels exhibit a "looping" with a lack of congestion (redness due to being engorged with an extra amount of blood). Limbal congestion is exhibited as vessel dilatation without vessel looping. Early neovascularization demonstrates limbal congestion with new vessel growth of less than 1 mm into the cornea, while neovascularization extends more than 1 mm into the cornea (see Chapter 10).

In order to maintain the proper relationship between the contact lens and the cornea, oxygen must be able to flow through the lens. Oxygen permeability (Dk) describes the permeability of a material to various gases such as oxygen. Oxygen transmissibility (Dk/L) relates the Dk value to the material based on the thickness (L) of the contact lens, thus describing the oxygen permeability at the contact's geometric center.[3, 4] To prevent corneal edema, certain levels of oxygen transmissibility through the contact lens must be achieved. The epithelium requires a Dk/L of 64.

The ability of a contact lens to allow oxygen transmission across the lens surface and deliver it to the cornea in a similar level to that of an eye without a contact lens is called the equivalent oxygen percent (EOP). In other words, EOP is the percentage of oxygen delivered to the cornea without a lens (atmospheric) versus the amount of oxygen delivered to the cornea with a contact lens acting as a barrier. Normal atmospheric air has an oxygen level of 21%. The oxygen requirements of the cornea, in order to avoid hypoxia, will vary between 5% and 10%. At 5% oxygen, the normal cornea will swell about 2%. At 8% oxygen, the cornea will swell about 1%. The normal cornea will tend to swell approximately 4% when the eye is closed (as during sleep); however, this can be substantially higher if extended or flexible wear contact lenses are worn during sleep.

Corneal Measurements; Understanding the Corneal Contour

It was traditionally thought that the cornea was composed of several sets of spheres. (A sphere is a geometric figure with an equal radius to all points from a fixed central point.) Recent technology has provided a better understanding of corneal shape. These technologies have defined the cornea as an aspheric surface having a steeper central area and progressing flatter periphery.

As it pertains to contact lens design, it is convenient to describe the cornea as two spherical zones (Figure 1-1). The first zone is the central sphere of the cornea, referred to as the corneal cap. The center, or optic zone, of the contact lens is designed to conform to the corneal cap. The second corneal zone is the flatter periphery, the area between the corneal cap and the limbus. The contact len's peripheral curve is designed to contour this zone.

In order to match the curve of the contact lens to the curve of the cornea, it is best to obtain some type of corneal measurement. There are several ways to do this, which are described in the following paragraphs.

OptT

Keratometry

The keratometer has long been the standard in measuring corneal curvature. There are several disadvantages associated with the keratometer. It is time-consuming with an inherent error rate

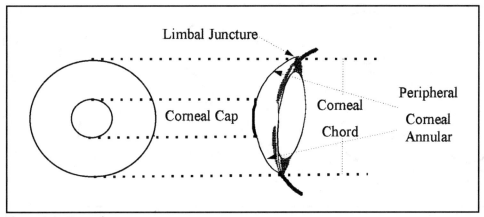

Figure 1-1. Corneal zones.

due to operator difficulties. The major disadvantage is that the keratometric measure is limited to the corneal cap. The mires are designed to evaluate the center of the corneal cap, limiting the measure to approximately 1.5 mm (reflections projected onto the cornea). This is only 8% of the corneal surface. Additionally, most instruments allow for the collection of only four data points, which is considered statistically insignificant. Still, the keratometer is considered adequate to measure the curvature of the cornea or any convex or concave surface.

The basic method for proper keratometric use is as follows:

1) Focus the ocular eyepiece by viewing the internal cross hair against a white piece of paper. Slowly adjust the eyepiece from its most plus position (where the cross hair will be blurred) toward the minus. At the point of best clarity, stop. Note this setting for future use.

2) The keratometer should be calibrated prior to use. The calibration is accomplished by measuring a steel ball of a known curvature. (Most commonly, the balls are 40.50 D, 42.50 D, and 44.75 D. They are attached to the keratometer with a magnetic mount.) If the measurements are inaccurate, follow the instrument's instruction manual to adjust the drum settings. (For more details, see Basic Bookshelf title *Instrumentation for Eyecare Paraprofessionals*.)

3) The second step is to align the keratometer with the patient's eye. Occlude the non-examined eye. Align the scope by placing a light into the ocular so that it shines down the keratometer tube and is projected onto the patient's cornea. Adjust the vertical and horizontal position of the instrument until the projected light is well-centered on the cornea.

4) Next, bring the mires into focus with the focusing knob. Then adjust the vertical and horizontal knobs to bring the mires into close alignment (Figure 1-2A).

5) The axis is identified by turning the keratometer tube until the "+" and "−" images (attached to the mire circle) are aligned.

6) Once the axis is identified, the horizontal and vertical knobs are fine-tuned until the "+" and "−" mires are overlapping (Figure 1-2B).

7) Make note of the readings on the scales. Commonly, the readings are noted as horizontal diopters at the horizontal meridian/vertical diopters at the vertical meridian. This may be followed by a calculation of the number of cylinder diopters present and a comment about the mire quality.

For example: 43.00 x 180 / 45.00 x 90, -2.00 diopters of cylinder (DC) x 180, Mires are clear and round.

For irregular corneas, treat each meridian separately, adjusting horizontal and then vertical.

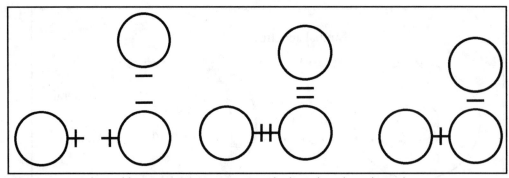

Figure 1-2A. Spherical keratometric mires: separated, aligned, and overlapped.

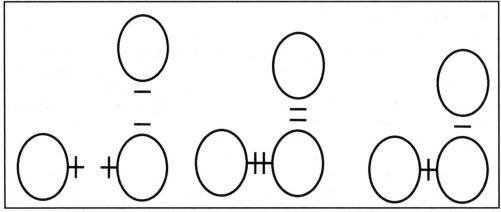

Figure 1-2B. Toric keratometric mires: separated, aligned, and overlapped.

8) Extending the range of the keratometer—The corneal measures may be excessively flat or steep, thereby exceeding the scales of the keratometer. If this occurs, tape a +1.25 (steeper) or -1.00 (flatter) trial lens onto the face of the keratometer without blocking the "+" or "–" extensions of the mire. Measure the cornea again and consult a conversion chart for the exact value (see Appendix). A +1.25 lens adds approximately 8 diopters to the measurement. A -1.00 lens subtracts about 8 diopters.

Computer Assisted Corneal Topography

Computer Assisted Corneal Topography (CACT) utilizes an image of concentric rings that is projected onto the cornea. CACT involves a video image capture system that allows for computer processing via a series of software applications. The data is processed via a series of algorithms (software applications) that will generate a series of qualitative descriptors. These descriptors are used to generate a colored map of the corneal surface. The sensitivity of the system depends on the proximity of the ring images to the cornea as well as the number of rings that can be projected. A variety of colorful topographic maps can be generated from keratometric and radius of curvature values (Table 1-1). The maps have specific shapes that are defined as "normal, astigmatic, or diseased." These maps will appear as symmetric to highly irregular, and are described as round, oval, symmetric or asymmetric bow tie, or irregular (amorphic) (Figure 1-3 and Table 1-2).

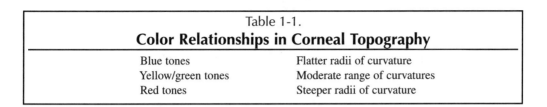

Table 1-1. Color Relationships in Corneal Topography	
Blue tones	Flatter radii of curvature
Yellow/green tones	Moderate range of curvatures
Red tones	Steeper radii of curvature

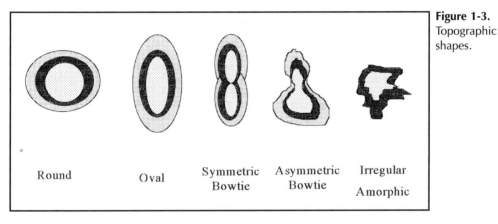

Figure 1-3. Topographic shapes.

Round   Oval   Symmetric Bowtie   Asymmetric Bowtie   Irregular Amorphic

Table 1-2. Implications of Corneal Topographic Shapes	
Round	Spherical
Oval	Low astigmatism (-0.25 to -0.75)
Symmetric bow tie	Moderate to high astigmatism
Asymmetric bow tie	High to irregular astigmatism or underlying clinical pathology (ie, keratoconus, pellucid, rigid gas permeable lens warping, etc)
Irregular or amorphic	Severe corneal distortion from disease, trauma, or surgery

Newer software applications allow the clinician to design hydrophilic and rigid lens for the patient prior to diagnostic lens insertion. These software applications will prove to be advantageous when designing lenses, reducing valuable chair time and refitting.

References

1. Brennan NA, Effron N, Bruce AS, Duldig DI, Russo NJ. Dehydration of hydrogel lenses: environmental influences during normal wear. *American Journal of Optometry and Physiological Optics.* 1998;65(4):277-281.

2. Bruce AS, Brennan NA. Clinical observations of the post-lens tear film during the first hour of hydrogel lens wear. *International Contact Lens Clinic.* October 1988;15(10):304-310.

3. McMonnies CW. Key questions in a dry eye history. *J Am Optom Assoc.* July 1986;57(7):512-517.

4. McMonnies CW, Ho A. Patient history in screening for dry eye conditions. *J Am Optom Assoc.* April 1987;58(4):296-301.

Chapter 2

Contact Lens Design, Parameters, and Optics

- The base curve (BC) establishes the core fit of the contact lens and acts as the template for the peripheral curve system.

- Rigid and hydrophilic lenses are designed as "ultra thin" to enhance oxygen permeability (referred to as Dk/L) to the central cornea.

- The contour of the lens edge will have a direct interaction with the lid, cornea, and conjunctiva to stabilize the lens on the eye, assist with lens movement, and optimize tear exchange.

- The optic zone diameter (OZD) has a major influence on the lens power, overall dimensions, and central fit.

- The general rule is that smaller OZDs will act flatter and larger diameters will act steeper.

- Blending is a process of polishing the juncture points smooth to reduce the prismatic effect and enhance comfort.

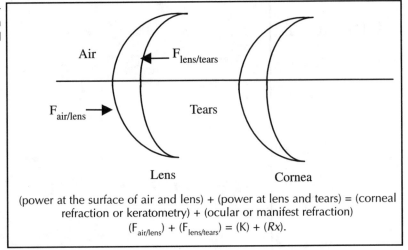

Figure 2-1. Relationship between contact lens and cornea.

Air

$F_{lens/tears}$

$F_{air/lens}$

Tears

Lens

Cornea

(power at the surface of air and lens) + (power at lens and tears) = (corneal refraction or keratometry) + (ocular or manifest refraction)

$$(F_{air/lens}) + (F_{lens/tears}) = (K) + (Rx).$$

When early contact lens pioneers started to work with the concept of placing a lens on the eye, they realized that the eye's anatomical structure was the first factor that needed to be addressed (Figure 2-1). Lens fitting objectives developed which required the lens to conform to the ocular surface without traumatizing the tissue, while yielding adequate vision.

Lens Parameters

OptT

Safety, comfort, and vision are accomplished by understanding contact lens parameters and their relationship to anterior segment anatomy. Contact lens parameters establish a blueprint for lens design. There are a multitude of parameters for hard, rigid, and soft (hydrophilic) contact lenses (Table 2-1). Each individual parameter can have a dramatic effect on the final contact lens-cornea relationship.

OptA

Base Curve

OptA

The base curve (BC) can also be referred to as the central posterior curve (CPC) or optic zone radius (OZR). The BC is the primary curve of the contact lens that is designed to match the central corneal contour and shape. The BC establishes the core fit of the contact lens and acts as the template for the peripheral curve (PCR) system. Keratometric or topographic measures are generally used to determine the CPC, specified in millimeters or diopters.

Fitting a rigid lens to the flattest keratometric value is called "fitting on K," or an "alignment" fit. Fitting flatter than the flat keratometric value will yield a "bearing" or "touch" effect on the central cornea, while fitting steeper than the flat keratometric value will yield a "clearance" effect. CPCs can also fit flatter than the flattest keratometric value in each meridian, as with a toric lens design for astigmatism.

When fitting soft (hydrophilic) lenses, the BC is selected to compensate for the lens's ability to conform to the cornea. The BC for hydrophilic lenses is specified as steep (8.0 to 8.3 mm), median (8.4 to 8.8 mm), or flat (8.9 to 9.1 mm).

Table 2-1.
Contact Lens Parameters

Parameter	Corneal/Contact Lens Relation
BC or CPC in diopters or millimeters	Primary curve of the contact to match the central corneal contour and shape. The BC establishes the core fit of the contact lens and establishes the base for the PCR system.
Power (P) or Diopters of sphere (DS), Diopters of cylinder (DC), and Axis (x)	The vertex corrected diopteric value of the contact lens. $$F = \{ F_1 - (L_c F_1 / n)\} + F_2$$ F_1 = back vertex power $= (1 - n) / r_1$ F_2 = front surface power $= (1 - n) / r_2$ r_1 = radius of front focal r_2 = radius of back focal (or F = power) L_c = lens thickness n = index of refraction for the material
Overall Diameter (D) in millimeters	Linear measure from lens edge to lens edge, respecting the overall corneal diameter in the horizontal, vertical, and oblique.
Center Thickness (L or CT) in millimeters	The thickness in the geometric center of the contact lens which will determine the stability or prevention of flexure and the oxygen permeability of the material.
Edge Thickness/Profile (ET) in millimeters	Thickness/profile at the edge of the lens that will affect lid and conjunctival relationships.
Optical Zone Diameter (OZD) in millimeters	The optical portion of the lens surrounding the geometric center. This area influences power and fit. It establishes the base measure for overall diameter and the PCR widths.
Posterior PCR System in millimeters	Additional paracentral curves which will establish the proper alignment to the peripheral cornea and conjunctiva, provide tear reservoir, and allow for the proper lens movement in relation to lid interaction.
Transition zones or Blends	Point or juncture between each posterior curve, CPC, and posterior PCR system.
Central Anterior Curve (CAC)	Establishes the front vertex power of the lens.
Anterior Optical Zone (AOZ) or Optical Cap	Encompasses the front surface of the contact. It may incorporate a toric (astigmatic) correction.
Lens Mass	Weight of the contact lens in milligrams.
Aspheric (non spherical surface) = Eccentricity (e)	Deviation from a circular path established by a series of conical sections, such as an ellipse, parabola, or hyperbola. Establishes a front and back surface curvature to contour the corneal surface center to periphery.
Material	Hard (PMMA), Rigid Gas Permeable, Hydrophilic—Hydrogel.
Fenestration	Holes drilled through the lens surface to increase tear fluid exchange.
Lenticulation or Carrier	Added or reduced peripheral mass to assist in lens positioning and lid interaction.
Chord	The distance from edge to edge of the contact lens or the diameter of the optic zone.
Sagitta	The distance between a point on the lens surface and the midpoint of the chord.

When changing the BC of a lens, the lens power must also be adjusted according to the following rules:

1) Flatter add plus (FAP): When flattening the BC, plus power is added to the lens.

2) Steeper add minus (SAM): When steepening the BC, minus power is added to the lens.

3) For each 0.05 mm change in BC, 0.25 diopters of power is added or subtracted based on the FAP/SAM criteria.

(These rules do not apply to soft hydrophilic contact lens since they conform to the corneal surface.)

Other Parameters

Sagittal Depth

Sagittal depth (or vertical height) is the measure from the posterior lens surface intersecting the midpoint of the chord dimension. The chord is the distance from one edge to the other, or the diameter. The steeper the BC measure, the greater the radius or sagitta. In contrast, the flatter the BC, the shorter the radius or sagitta (Figure 2-2).

Overall Diameter

The Overall Diameter (D) is a linear measure of the lens from edge to edge. It is the measure of the greatest distance across the outside of the lens. A hydrophilic lens will have an overall lens diameter of approximately 1 to 1.5 mm larger than the visible iris diameter. Lens diameters for hydrophilic lenses are larger than those available for rigid lenses, ranging from 12.5 mm (mini) to 16 mm (scleral lens design). The diameters most commonly used for hydrophilic lenses range between 13.8 to 14.5 mm.

A rigid lens will have a lens diameter 1.0 to 1.5 mm smaller than the visible iris diameter. Rigid gas permeable lenses are fit within the corneal dimensions, averaging 8.5 to 10 mm. The lens diameter for rigid lenses is based on the desired fitting relationship (see Chapter 5).

Center Thickness

Center Thickness (L or CT) is the thickness in the geometric center of the contact lens. This determines both oxygen permeability and lens stability. (The lack of lens stability is also referred to as flexure.) The CT of a lens plays an integral role in both the physiological relationship and mechanical stability of the contact lens.

Lenses should be as thin as possible in order to maintain optimal oxygen permeation. A thin lens will foster better tear exchange while reducing the potential for corneal edema, optimizing comfort, and decreasing lens awareness. If lenses are excessively thin, there is more chance for flexure, which will distort the lens optics. Flexure will mimic a steep lens fit, create tear stasis, and trap debris, which will cause corneal distortion. The CT of the lens can be specified by the designer, based on the manufacturer's templates and proper specifications.

Hydrophilic lenses are "ultra-thin," averaging 0.04 to 0.11 mm depending on the material, water content, and potential wear schedule. CT and water content are the two major factors in determining if a contact lens can be approved for daily and/or extended wear. A hydrophilic lens is considered extended wear for a maximum of 6 nights and 7 days (then is to be removed and cleansed or discarded) with parameters of 38% water and 0.03 to 0.07 mm CT. Extended wear hydrophilic lenses can also be 55% water with a CT of 0.08 to 0.10 mm. These specifications are designed to prevent corneal compromise.

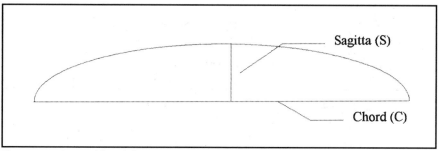

Figure 2-2. Sagitta/chord dimensions.

The CT of rigid gas permeable lenses can vary based on the material and manufacturing. These lenses are "ultra-thin" to enhance oxygen permeability (referred to as the Dk/L) to the central cornea. The CT will also affect the final lens profile and the edge thickness. Finally, the CT assists in the long-term stability of the lens. It must have sufficient thickness to avoid flexure and warping. Rigid lenses are fabricated with thicknesses ranging from 0.09 mm (minus) to 0.50 mm (high plus), averaging from 0.10 to 0.15 mm.

Lens power will also effect the final center thickness. A plus lens will be thicker centrally and thinner peripherally. This may lead to a lower Dk/L value unless compensated for by using a higher Dk lens material. The thicker center will shift the center of gravity anteriorly, forcing the lens to decenter (displace from the central cornea) inferiorly. Additionally, a plus lens may have a proportionally thin edge design. If excessively thin, the designer may need to incorporate a "minus lenticular design."

Lenticulation is a process of adding bulk to the periphery of a plus lens or reducing the mass of a minus lens. Lenticulation is generally not considered until a lens power reaches 64.00 diopters. When a lens power exceeds ±4.00 diopters, a minus lens requires a decrease in edge thickness while a plus lens requires an increase in the edge thickness. An increase in edge thickness is called a minus lenticular (myoflange) while a decrease in edge thickness is called a plus lenticular (hyperflange). Alternately, a thick lens edge can be polished incorporating a CN bevel or anterior peripheral tapering to round and smooth the lens edge (see Chapter 9, Lens Verification and Modification Techniques).

Lens diameter can also effect the CT. The smaller the lens diameter is, the thinner the lens that can be fabricated.

Edges

The edge thickness (ET) or edge profile is the thickness at the edge of the lens that comes into direct contact with the cornea and/or conjunctiva. When designing the contact lens, the ET should be thin, approximately 0.08 mm for rigid lenses and 0.03 mm for hydrophilic lenses. The profile should be rounded in order to avoid corneal or conjunctival chafing and injury. The contour of the lens edge will have direct interaction with the lid to either stabilize the lens on the eye and/or to assist with lens movement.

An alignment fit has an edge that requires that the lid and lens edge have a mutually respectful relationship. A palpebral aperture fit (fits between the lids) requires a thin edge profile in order to avoid excessive lid interaction. (This allows the lens to settle centrally on the cornea, avoiding lid adherence.)

The edge design of hydrophilic contact lens requires the edge profile to be round and thin in order to enhance conjunctival relationships.

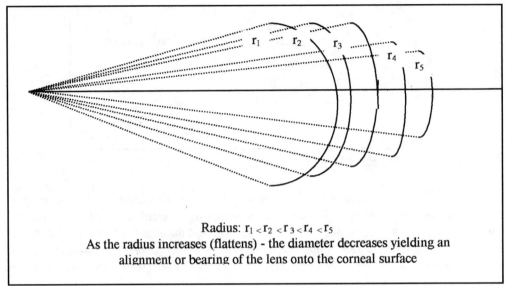

Radius: $r_1 < r_2 < r_3 < r_4 < r_5$
As the radius increases (flattens) - the diameter decreases yielding an
alignment or bearing of the lens onto the corneal surface

Figure 2-3. Effects of OZD on the central radius of curvature.

Optic Zone

The optic zone diameter (OZD) runs across the optical portion of the lens surrounding the geometric center. It is also the linear dimension of the posterior optical radius. The OZD can be either spherical or oval based on the shape of the cornea. There are two optic zones, the anterior (AOZD) and the posterior (POZD). The OZD has a major influence on the lens power, overall dimensions, and the central fit. It establishes the base measure for the overall diameter and the PCR widths. (The overall diameter is calculated by adding the PCR widths to the OZD.) If the optic zone is decreased it will mimic a minor flattening effect on the overall fit of the lens.

The optic zone has a dramatic effect on fit due to its relation to the anterior corneal surface (Figure 2-3). When adjusting the lens fit, the OZD is increased if the desired effect is to steepen the lens. In contrast, the diameter can be decreased if the desired effect is to flatten the lens. As the OZD is adjusted, the BC needs to be properly modified using a 0.05 mm = 0.25 diopters ratio. The general rule is that smaller OZDs will act flatter and larger diameters will act steeper.

The OZD should be large enough as not to impinge on the pupillary margin when the pupil is fully dilated (Table 2-2). The OZD should be small enough to maintain a trace to minimal clearance of the anterior corneal surface. When determining the OZD, the pupil diameter needs to be judged at mid- to full-dilation (without dilating drops). A larger pupil requires an OZD in order to avoid visual problems such as flare.

Flare and distortion are usually caused by the prismatic effect at the first juncture between the optic zone and the secondary curve (SCR). A general rule of thumb is to design an optic zone equal to, or slightly greater than, the millimeter value of the BC.

Curve Systems

The posterior PCR system is the set of paracentral curves that establish an alignment to the peripheral cornea and conjunctiva. The PCR system is a series of concentric curves designed to follow the natural contour of the cornea from the immediate paracentral region (ie, the central 6 to 7 mm) to the extreme periphery. The PCR system is designed to complement the peripheral

Table 2-2. Optic Zone Diameter: Pupil and Keratometric Value Relations	
Small pupils and/or steeper CPC	OZD = CPC
Moderate pupils and/or moderate keratometric values	OZD = CPC + 0.1 to 0.2 mm
Large pupils and/or flatter keratometric values	OZD = CPC + 0.2 to 0.3 mm

cornea while reducing lens bearing. This will allow for an adequate tear reservoir exchange during blinking and proper lens movement without obstruction or resistance.

The PCR system can incorporate as many curves as necessary, limited only by the manufacturers' or laboratory's ability to fabricate each curve. A monocurve lens has no PCRs. A bicurve lens has a CPC and an SCR specified as radius of curvature and width. A tricurve has a CPC, an SCR, and a PCR with specified radii of curvature and width. Finally, a tetracurve system incorporates a CPC, an SCR, an intermediate curve (ICR), and a PCR. The PCR radii and widths are designed to complement the peripheral corneal topography.

Hydrogel lenses follow the same philosophy of PCR system design. The goal is to create a vault over the limbal juncture, yielding a sufficient clearance to avoid hypoxia and neovascularization. Most hydrogel designs are limited to either a monocurve or bicurve design.

The transition zone or blends are defined as the point at where two posterior curves meet. If there is a significant difference between the two radii, the juncture will be sharp and will need to be smoothed. The juncture points inward towards the cornea. If the first juncture or transition is within the pupillary zone, the patient will likely complain about distortions and flare. To avoid these complaints, increase the optic zone and blend the junctures. (Blending is a process of polishing the juncture points smooth to reduce the prismatic effect.) If the blends are not properly tapered, the patient will complain of lens awareness and discomfort. Blends can be specified as light, medium, smooth, or heavy. A heavy blend makes the juncture between radii indistinguishable.

Water Content, Wetting Angle, and Elasticity

The water content (of soft lenses) is specified as low (38% or less), moderate (38% to 45%), or high (55% or greater). The water content is a factor in qualifying a lens for daily wear or extended wear use. Water content is also a critical factor in patient complaints pertaining to "dry eye" symptoms.

Lenses have been demonstrated to lose approximately 6% to 10% of their water content within the first 6 hours of wear. When the lens dehydrates, it will tend to steepen and may become tighter on the eye. The tightness may be associated with additional patient complaints of difficult lens removal, blurred vision, and ocular redness.

The wetting angle defines the ability of moisture to spread evenly over the lens surface. This is important in maintaining hydration of the lens. The wetting angle is measured as the tangent to the surface of a water droplet on a solid surface (Figure 2-4). The most favorable wetting angle would be 180. Partial wetting is less than 90, and nonwetting is greater than 90.

The modulus of elasticity defines the inherent flexibility of the material. Rigid lenses will maintain a low modulus of elasticity or inflexibility while hydrogel lenses will have a high modulus of elasticity. The elasticity of a lens is a direct chemical relationship associated with the amount of acrylate or methylarylate in the material's polymer backbone. The degree of elasticity is based on the polymerization process for the material (see next section).

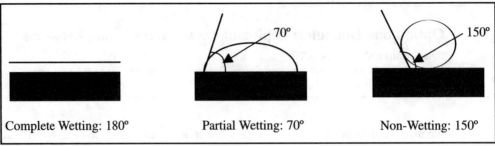

Complete Wetting: 180° Partial Wetting: 70° Non-Wetting: 150°

Figure 2-4. Wetting angle.

Figure 2-5. Swell factors and dimensions.

Swell factor = wet dimensions/dry dimensions

Dimensions: CT, BC, longitudinal expansion, radial expansion, power

Power factor = dry power/wet power

Radius = $(S_1)^2/S_2$

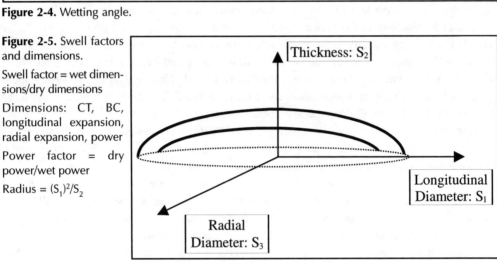

Swell Factor

Lathe cut and dry cast molded lenses mimic rigid gas permeable lenses during manufacturing. After the lens is fabricated, it is placed into saline for hydration, at which time the lens polymer "swells." From the rigid to the hydrated state a hydration, or swell factor, can be applied (Figure 2-5). Generally, a final BC for a hydrogel lens will be approximately 1.3 to 1.4 mm greater than the BC in the dehydrated state. This factor can be applied to BC selection for hydrogel lenses. Simply add 1.3 mm to the flat keratometric reading to approximate the hydrogel BC of choice. For example: 7.5 mm (45) flat keratometry + 1.3 mm would equal an 8.8 mm hydrophilic BC selection.

Lens Fabrication

Polymers are defined as plastics of "many parts." A monomer, or "single part," is the basic component or unit of the polymer. Monomers are linked into a consistent, repeating chain by a process called polymerization. Polymers used in lens making are in liquid or solid-rod form. Fabrication processes include spin cast molding, dry cast molding, and lathe cutting.

Spin cast molding is a process where a liquid monomer (thermoplastic) is placed into a concave mold that is spun at a high velocity, using centrifugal force to spread the monomer. The front curve is predetermined by the cast while the back curve is aspheric. (The amount of asphericity is determined by the velocity of the spinning process.) The material is then polymerized by exposure to ultraviolet light into a dry form and hydrated in normal saline. Spin cast lenses are the least expensive to manufacture, but have slightly steeper fitting characteristics.

In dry cast molding, the monomer is placed into a front concave mold (female) of a specific curve. Compressing a back surface (male) mold into the female mold creates the BC. The monomer spreads between the front and back mold. The mold is placed into a heat oven, forming a "dry" lens. The lens is removed from the mold and hydrated in normal saline. This is a favorable method for hydrogel manufacturing as it allows for a cost efficient and customized lens design.

The lathe cut process, used with rigid and hydrogel lenses, uses a monomer rod. The monomer rod is cut into buttons. The buttons are placed on a lathe to cut either the back and/or front surface of the lens. The lathe cutter utilizes diamond blades for precision cutting. This allows for a variety of shapes as well as for thicknesses, PCRs, and diameters. Until recently, this was considered an inefficient method due to limitations and inconsistencies in mass production. Recently, however, with the introduction of new technology, lenses can be easily produced in mass volume with a very high level of reproducibility and at a moderate cost.

Aspheric Lens Design

An aspheric design has a non-spherical surface, which assumes that the cornea is an ellipse. The back surface of the lens has a specified eccentricity (e) that describes the progressively flattening contour of the lens. As the e value increases, this implies that the surface is flattening. The cornea is aspheric, but not in a continuously symmetric fashion. The asphericity of the contact lens will vary in each meridian, consistent with the corneal astigmatism (CA). An aspheric lens would be a preferred design for low cylinders, but not for moderate to higher cylinders. (For higher cylinders, a toric design is required.)

The aspheric design is classified into three categories:

- Spherical posterior optic zone with aspheric periphery: used for flatter corneas with a continuously flatter periphery.
- Aspheric posterior optic zone with aspheric periphery: used for steeper corneas with a continuously steeper periphery.
- Bispheric (front and back surfaces): used for special fitting and optical requirements such as multifocal or astigmatic designs.

Aspheric lenses have several uses related to the optical characteristics of the lens. Aspheric lenses increase the efficiency of lens centration due to a slightly steeper cornea/lens relation. This will assist in the correction of low to moderate cylinders. The ability of the lens to center adequately and consistently will also decrease lens awareness and increase comfort.

The lens mass or weight affects such factors as the specific gravity of the material, lens power, and overall design requirements. The lens mass is measurable in milligrams as dry or wet weight depending on whether the material is rigid or hydrogel. The lens mass is directly proportional to the CT, which in turn will affect lens centration. Any increase in lens mass will cause the lens to decenter inferiorly and mimic a steep lens fit. When lenses appear to decenter inferiorly, the designer should consider a CT reduction. If a lens decenters superiorly or has excessive lid interaction, the designer should consider an increase in the CT or the addition of prism to increase the lens mass.

Contact Lens Optics

The contact lens is actually a miniature spectacle lens. Because of its contact with the eye, there are additional optical effects that must be considered. Contact lenses vary in many aspects

Figure 2-6. Lensometer stop supports the contact lens.

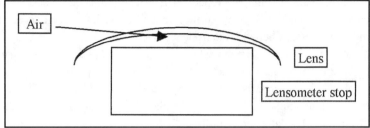

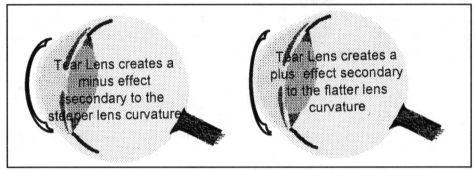

Figure 2-7. Tear lens effect secondary to lens curvature.

from spectacle lenses due to thickness, vertex distance (or effective power), magnification effects, prismatic effects, field of view, and optical aberrations. Contact lenses also have significant visual effects in terms of changes to accommodative demand.

Front vertex or back vertex power readings can be taken by standard lensometry to determine the lens power. (Present convention is to read back vertex power.) This is done by placing the back surface of the contact lens onto the lensometer stop so that the front surface is facing the examiner (Figure 2-6). The power of the contact lens is specified in diopters of sphere and cylinder. (See also Chapter 9, Lens Verification and Modification Techniques.)

The BC of the contact lens is specified by the concave surface. The BC is designed to establish alignment or minimal clearance and to allow the lens to be properly supported by the cornea without adversely effecting comfort or physiology. The BC establishes the basic lens design after which the additional lens parameters are incorporated.

The power effect of the contact lens on the eye is a combination of the lens and the tear film (Figure 2-7). This creates a dynamic system or liquid lens power. If the lens is in perfect alignment or is bearing onto the cornea, the tear layer will have minimal effect on the contact lens power. However, if the lens demonstrates a degree of clearance, the tear film *will* have a power effect on the cornea/tear/lens system. Since a rigid lens maintains its shape, it is assumed there will always be a tear layer effect. However, with soft or hydrogel lenses the tear layer is negated due to the lack of lens rigidity and the material's ability to contour to the corneal surface. (The tear layer which does exist is minute and demonstrates no power effect.)

The final power effect to be considered is the *effective power*. This is the adjustment in lens power from spectacle plane to corneal plane. If a lens is moved into a closer proximity to the cornea, the power will need to be increased by adding plus. This will allow the image to remain focused on the fovea. If power is not increased, the image will be displaced beyond the fovea, leaving the patient undercorrected. If the lens is moved away from the cornea, power needs to be reduced by adding minus. An acronym for this effect is CAP: Closer Add Plus. Effectivity becomes appreciable in calculations at powers greater than ±4.00 diopters.

For example: A spectacle presentation of -6.00 – 1.00 x 180, 44/45 at 90 or -1.00 x 180.

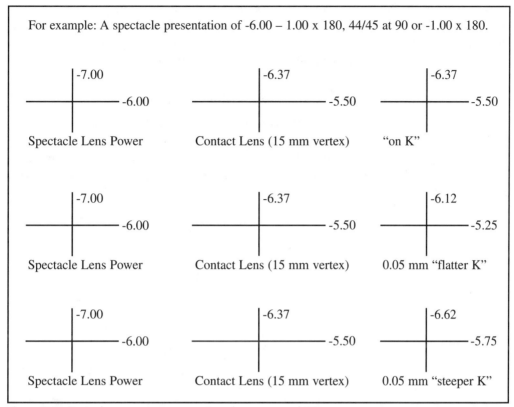

Figure 2-8. Optical cross power corrections for vertex and BC.

An over-refraction (over-refractometry) is the process of power refinement in contact lens fitting. The over-refraction may be performed either with the phoropter or with a hand-held trial lens. The over-refraction is most effective when the contact lens is close to the desired final power. If the over-refraction power is greater than ±4.00 diopters, a vertex correction for the over-refraction power needs to be incorporated into the final lens prescription.

Astigmatism is the presence of two separate power meridians on the optical surface that in turn create two points of focus. There are two forms of astigmatism that will effect the final contact lens design: corneal and lenticular.

CA is measured by standard keratometry or topography. Lenticular astigmatism (astigmatism caused by irregular curvature of the crystalline lens) is measured by subjective or manifest refraction. (Residual astigmatic power is the difference between the refractive cylinder and the keratometric cylinder.)

Uncorrected CA occurs more frequently when a rigid lens is fit steeper than the flattest keratometric reading. Due to the steep relation between the cornea and the lens, a tear layer effect will be manifested. "Fitting on K" will negate much of the tear layer power effect.

Many patients can tolerate an uncorrected 0.50 DC against-the-rule or oblique cylinder or a maximum of 0.75 DC with-the-rule cylinder.

Astigmatic over-refractions are easily incorporated into power adjustments for rigid or hard lenses. This is accomplished by treating the over-refraction as an independent lens and adding it to the contact lens power via an optical cross (Figure 2-8). Vertex or effectivity should be considered first. Then a simple addition is completed. The astigmatic over-refraction implies two things.

First, it could imply that the lens is not in proper alignment with the cornea, thereby exhibiting uncorrected CA (suggesting that a back toric lens needs to be fit). Second, it could imply that internal astigmatism has not been corrected (requiring a front toric lens). Be sure to rule out lens flexure or warping, which would require a thicker lens design and/or lens replacement.

Accommodative Effects Associated with Contact Lenses

Accommodation is the action of the ciliary muscle to change the shape of the crystalline lens. With the use of contact lenses, myopes will have a greater demand on accommodation due to the absence of base-out prism that is normally present in their spectacles. Hyperopic accommodative demand is slightly lessened in contact lenses due to the increase in plus power associated with vertex correction.

Chapter 3

Patient Selection and Examination Procedures

OptT

KEY POINTS

- The first contact person(s) (the office staff) sets the tone for the examination and the aftercare.

- A survey should be used to collect pertinent information regarding health (systemic and ocular), occupation, hobbies, previous eyecare and/or correction, contact lens use (if any), and insurance coverage.

- The psychological and motivational aspects of contact lens wear are the most important factors in long-term success.

- A patient who is verbally interactive and able to reason is never too young for contact lenses. The limiting factor is the patient's ability to understand the need to follow a maintenance schedule or to comply with a set wearing and care schedule without deviation.

- The cylinder sensitivity test determines the patient's appreciation for uncorrected astigmatism in spectacles and contact lenses.

- By interrelating the patient's needs with clinical experience and knowledge, the choice of contact lens design and material becomes streamlined.

It is a rarity that a patient cannot be fit with contact lenses. Often, it is improper selection or questioning of a patient that discourages a new fit. Patient selection for contact lenses is largely based on motivation. If the motivation exists, then the door is open. Once the door is open, the clinician must ask the proper questions to identify the variety of contact lens options that will best meet the needs of the patient. Such needs involve vision, health, and desired use of contact lenses.

The Phone Interview

During the initial phone interview, the staff member can offer information pertaining to contact lenses. He or she can inquire whether the patient is presently wearing, or is interested in contact lenses. If the patient already wears contact lenses, the interviewer can offer information pertaining to new products and gather information pertaining to present lens use. ("When you come in, you may want to ask the doctor if you are a candidate for X, Y, Z, product.") If the caller is not a contact lens wearer, the interviewer should ask: "Have you ever worn contact lenses, or are you interested in contact lenses?" If yes, say, "When you see the doctor, you may want to ask about some of the new contact lens options that may work well for you."

The In-Office Interview

The second part of the patient interview takes place in the office. Once the patient arrives, a survey should be used to collect pertinent information regarding health (systemic and ocular), occupation, hobbies, previous eyecare and/or correction, contact lens use (if any), and insurance coverage. The information gathered in the survey will allow the technical staff and the doctor to immediately familiarize themselves with the patient's needs and concerns (Table 3-1). This facilitates communication and allows for a more efficient examination. The survey also gives personal information that will allow social conversation, making the patient feel more comfortable in the new environment.

The technician/doctor-patient interview follows a review of the survey. During the patient interview the patient should be encouraged to give his or her concerns and reasons for the visit. The examiner should then repeat the chief complaint and initiate further questioning. (Examples of additional questions include onset, frequency, severity, location, one or both eyes, and accompanying ocular and/or systemic associations, etc.) After the chief concern is addressed, a general review of the medical and ocular history should follow. This includes asking whether or not the patient is wearing or has ever worn contact lenses, as well as whether or not he or she is interested in trying them now. (For a complete text on history taking, see *The Complete Guide to Ocular History Taking* by Jan Ledford.)

The survey (or interview) should identify specific occupational and avocational activities of the patient. Often, patients will have a variety of visual requirements based on their activities, such as safety and/or sports eyewear, or computer and occupational eyewear. It is advantageous to further question the patient about occupational safety requirements due to specific Occupational Safety and Health Administration (OSHA) regulations. Such regulations may prohibit the use of contact lenses.

If the patient is interested in contact lenses, investigate the patient's psychological motivation and type of previous vision correction. What is the patient's goal for the use of contact lenses: part time, full time, daily, flexible, or extended wear? What was his or her previous experience

Table 3-1.
Indications and Contraindications for Contact Lenses

Indications for Contact Lenses	Contraindications of Contact Lenses
Cosmesis	Age
Refractive	Hygiene problems
Improvement of visual quality (ie,high refractive errors, aphakia, irregular astigmatism, postoperative)	Hypersensitivity reactions (care product concern)
Corneal disease (ie, keratoconus, pellucid, dystrophies, scar, trauma)	Aphakia and/or glaucoma with blebs
Binocular vision (ie, anisometropia, nystagmus, amblyopia, aniseikonia)	Moderate to severe dry eye (circumvented with punctal occlusion or lubricant therapy)
Occupational requirements	Immuno-suppression
Sports activity: enhanced peripheral field of vision	Thyroid disease (Hypothyroidism: dryness, tear insufficiency; Hyperthyroidism: exophthalmos—exposure)
Social activity: cosmetics	Diabetes mellitus (healing problems—cellular fragility)
Therapeutic (ie, drug delivery, bandage, exposure protection)	Skin disorders (increased risk of ocular infection)
Low vision aid (ie, telescope or microscope—contact lens systems)	Neurological or retinal disease ie, CN 5/7 with related corneal hypothesia injury risk; however, may need a lens for therapeutic protection

with contact lenses? Has he or she been wearing spectacles only, if at all? Has he or she ever been fully corrected for the refractive error, or has the correction been reduced in the spectacle or contact lens correction? If the patient has worn contact lenses, were the lenses rigid, soft spheres, spherical equivalent power lens, or torics (and, if so, what design)?

Psychological Aspects of Patient Selection

The psychological and motivational aspects of contact lens wear are the most important factor to long-term success. There are inherent anxieties with all new things, particularly when it has a medical orientation. The clinician needs to be aware of the patient's apprehensions and present the options based on the patient's expressed motivation level. Motivation level can be characterized as: "No way," "I'm curious—but apprehensive," "I've thought about it," "I like my glasses, but..," "I will not be seen in glasses," and "I want to be able to see clearly all the time, even when I awake."

Motivation is directly related to the patient's "discomfort level," be it physical, psychological, or perceptual. Various motivators inspire a patient to inquire about contact lenses. These include:

- visual correction enhancement by reducing the use of spectacles
- cosmetic appearance of spectacles is less than desired
- alternate option to spectacle correction

- the patient's perception of handicap when the refractive error is uncorrected ("subjective blindness")

There are a few conditions in which a contact lens is required for a visual function or a visual handicap. These include keratoconus, aphakia, anisometropia, and degenerative myopia. In contrast, if a patient is psychologically "uncomfortable" with spectacles, he or she will not properly use them. Such a patient is an excellent candidate for contact lenses. This is often seen in adolescent and young adult populations due to the cosmetic appearance of spectacles.

The following exercise may be extremely helpful prior to lens placement. This technique will alert the fitter if the patient will be overly apprehensive about touching his or her own eye or is at ease with the concept. (If the patient cannot touch his or her own eye, it is best to send him or her home to practice the exercise prior to lens fitting.)

1) Ask the patient to wash his or her hands, explaining that some soap may contain oil, lanolin, or other additives that should not be used with contact lenses.

2) Without using a mirror, place the patient's thumb on the check and pull the lower eyelid down with the middle finger.

3) Place the patient's index finger (same hand) onto the white of the eye and lightly move it about. It will not hurt. (However, the eye might get mildly dry or irritated.)

Goals and Expectations

When interviewing the patient, ascertain the patient's motivation and goals. Goals can be defined as wear schedules plus occupational and avocational needs. It is vastly important, from a clinical viewpoint, to understand the goals of the patient as related to proper counseling as well as to selection of lens materials and care products.

For example:

- Does the patient require contact lenses for visual function? Is he or she visually handicapped without corrective eyewear?
- Will contact lenses improve the patient's visual performance at work, or in sports or hob-bies?
- Are contact lenses to be worn as part-time, daily, flexible, or extended wear?
- Is cosmesis the sole purpose of contact lenses?
- Is the responsibility level of the patient adequate to maintain contact lenses?

Maturity has always been a major question, particularly with children and young adults. These individuals often have the motivation but not the responsibility level. The fitter will need to make a judgment based on interaction with the patient, as well as a confidential interview with the parent when appropriate. Pediatric fitting not only requires the motivation of the patient, but more importantly the motivation of the parent or caretaker (see section on Pediatric Contact Lens Fitting, Chapter 12).

A patient who is verbally interactive and able to reason is rarely too young for contact lenses. The limiting factor is the patient's ability to understand the need to follow a maintenance, wear, and care schedule.

Preconceptions and Education

Preconceptions can inhibit a patient from inquiring about contact lenses. It is possible that the patient may have tried lenses two decades ago and had a "bad" experience. It is possible that another clinician told the patient that he or she could not wear contact lenses because of their pre-scription requirements (ie, astigmatism). It is the job of the staff and doctor to properly educate the patient on the possibility of the contact lens fit, both the positives and the negatives. Education (and re-education) of the patient is probably more difficult than clinical care.

The best patient is an educated patient. The patient should be encouraged to ask questions. The more that the patient understands the ramifications of his or her actions, the less the chance for mistakes and adverse effects.

Misconceptions that may negatively effect expectations are cost, handling and care, insertion and removal, cosmesis, and comfort. The use of itemized cost forms will assist in the financial discussion. Manufacturing technologies and intra-professional competition has reduced the cost of contact lenses to the same level as (if not less than) spectacles. Handling, care, comfort, and insertion and removal issues can be demonstrated and discussed. However, the patient's preconceived notions will not be disabled until a diagnostic trial lens is placed onto the eye. Once the lens is on the eye, the patient's anxiety and apprehensions are quickly replaced with "Why didn't I try this earlier?"

Advantages and Disadvantages

Education requires a review of the advantages and disadvantages of contact lenses. The advantages include:

- increased peripheral vision
- enhanced cosmetic appearance
- enhanced quality of vision due to lessened optical aberrations
- enhanced comfort, both physical and visual

However, there are several disadvantages with the use of contact lenses. These include:

- contact lenses are medical devices requiring care
- lenses need to be replaced more frequently than glasses, and are susceptible to coating and damage
- astigmatic correction may be incomplete
- due to lens dynamics, correctable vision may be more accurate and consistent with spectacles
- increased glare sensitivity
- possible increase in susceptibility to eye infections and/or inflammations

The Ocular Examination

The examination should follow the usual and customary standards set forth by the professional organizations and governing boards. These include visual acuities (with and without correction), visual field analysis, color vision, keratometry, refractometric measurement (dry and/or cyclo-plegic), binocular and accommodative functions, biomicroscopy, ophthalmoscopy, and intraocular pressures. For the prospective contact lens patient, additional testing should include refractometry at near, intermediate, and distance; astigmatic sensitivity (toric lens determination); measurements of iris/corneal diameters (vertical, horizontal, and oblique); corneal topography; pupil size and reactivity (lens and optic zone diameter); tear and blink function (ocular lens support); blink rate and lid tensions (lens movement/lid interaction); and palpebral aperture width (Figure 3-1).

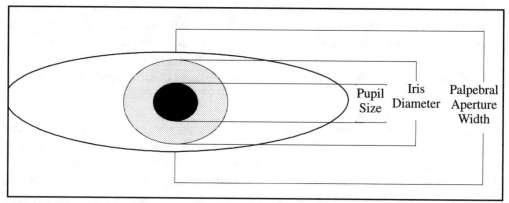

Figure 3-1. Ocular dimensions (to be measured in millimeters).

Refractometric Measurements

"Dry" (without cycloplegic drops) and "wet" (with cycloplegic drops) refractometric measurements should be performed. The dry refraction is performed to determine the optimal vision correction with respect to accommodation. In contrast, the wet refraction is used to determine the vision correction without accommodative influences.

The astigmatic cylinder and axis sensitivity need to be tested. This is called the "cylinder sensitivity test." First, the best correction should be placed into a trial frame or phoropter. Isolate the patient's best line of acuity and turn the axis dial clockwise and counterclockwise to the point of where the patient reports the first appreciable blur on either side. Next, return the axis to the dry refraction and then reduce the cylindrical correction to the point of first appreciable blur. (As cylinder is reduced, spherical compensation should be incorporated. Add 0.25 DS for each 0.50 DC subtracted.) At the point of cylindrical blur, add 0.25 DC to clear the image, and re-evaluate the axis sensitivity. This process determines the potential success of spherical equivalent and toric lens correction. Additionally, it demonstrates the potential "blur" that may occur with less than optimal vision. (The ultimate question is, if a minor blur or undercorrection exists with contact lenses, will it be visually tolerable?)

Presbyopic patients require an extra step. It is important to define the patient as a "true presbyope." A "true presbyope" accepts at least a +1.00 diopter add. An "incipient presbyope" is an individual who sees a benefit with additional plus at near, but does not *require* it at the time of the examination. In order to be a successful monovision or bifocal contact lens candidate, the patient must be able to tolerate a minor blur at distance and near. (The details of fitting presbyopes are covered in Chapter 11.)

Anterior Segment Examination

The primary concerns for the anterior segment are:
- tear function
- lid structure and closure
- corneal/conjunctival health
- lid aperture width
- pupil size
- corneal dimensions

Biomicroscopic examination of the lid, cornea, and conjunctival structures will determine the health of the eye and its ability to support a contact lens. The lids should be examined from gross and microscopic perspectives. Gross observation includes an extensive evaluation of lid anatomy and lid closure. Then scan the ocular anatomy for irregularities such as scars, lid flaking, redness, ecchymosis, epiphora, ectropion, entropion, growths, and so forth. Search for ocular surface defects such as pingueculae, pterygia, papillae, follicles, concretions, vascularization, and scars. (This is best done with a wide beam, moderate light intensity with the option of a diffusion filter.) The angle of the cornea is estimated with an optic section, after which the cornea is inspected. (For a complete discussion on biomicroscope technique, see Basic Bookshelf title *The Slit Lamp Primer*.)

OptA

Staining techniques should be done after the basic slit lamp examination. Sodium fluorescein (NaFl) and a cobalt (and/or yellow Wratten filter) is used to highlight areas of tissue defects. Tear break up time and tear meniscus are also measured with NaFl. (It is worth noting that some NaFl preparations may cause a reflexive tearing due to preservative irritations.) Later chapters will discuss corneal staining and ocular pathology associated with contact lenses.

Material and Lens Selection

Once the history is addressed and the patient is educated, the clinician needs to determine which material will best satisfy the ocular health and lifestyle needs of the patient. Allow the patient to have a part in the decision. There are several ways to satisfy comfort, visual, and wearing needs with various forms of contact lens designs and materials. (The advantages and disadvantages of various lenses will be discussed throughout the text.) A differential approach to lens selection is accomplished by charting the patient's needs against clinical information. This will reduce the decision to a choice of one or two lens designs and materials. When this is completed, the patient is ready to be fit.

Chapter 4

Fitting Hydrogel/Soft Contact Lenses

KEY POINTS

- Conventional or durable lenses are replaced after 6 months (or longer). Frequent replacement lenses have a life span of 1 to 3 months. Disposable lenses are worn either 1 day or 1 to 2 weeks.

- Daily wear lenses are removed each night; flexible wear are removed alternate nights; extended wear are removed after 6 nights.

- The water content of a material is classified as low to moderate (50% or less) or high (50% or higher).

- Hydrophilic lens diameters range from 12.5 to 16 mm, averaging between 13.8 to 14.5 mm.

- Spherical equivalence is calculated as half of the cylinder added to the spherical component of the prescription (with appropriate vertex correction).

- A lens evaluation is performed when the lens is inserted and after a 5-minute settling time. During the time of equilibration, the lens will start to dehydrate and grow steeper on the eye.

- A subjective survey of lens handling (including insertion and removal plus recognition of an inverted lens) and visual quality increase the potential success of the contact lens fit.

- The goal of a "best-fit scenario" is to find the best fit that is complemented by subjective acceptability for a variety of lens characteristics.

Introduction

To best understand the art of fitting soft contact lenses is to first understand the criteria of an optimal fitting scenario. Many techniques for lens evaluation have remained unchanged since the inception of hydrogel lenses. These evaluations include the characteristics of lens centration, corneal coverage, lens movement, tightness, physical comfort, visual acuity, and visual quality.

When fitting hydrogels, a diagnostic lens fit will expedite and optimize the results. Selection of the diagnostic lens is based on material and parameter availability. A diagnostic lens should meet the requirements predetermined by the subjective and objective measures in the pre-fitting examination. There are literally hundreds of hydrogel lenses available. Using diagnostic lens sets allow for ease of fitting without creating an excessive inventory.

The fitter should document the lens fitting characteristics that are consistent and reproducible. An optimal fit is well-positioned, centered, and moves well without hesitation (more on this later). A more precise method is to describe the specific characteristics in detail, such as lens position in primary, upward, and lateral gaze; decentration; tightness; surface quality; and so forth.

Classification by Replacement and Wear Schedules

Conventional or durable lenses have a life span greater than 6 months and are replaced (preferably) at intervals of no greater than 1 year (Table 4-1). Conventional lenses require a more effective care product system, such as peroxide.

Frequent replacement lenses have a life span of 1 to 3 months, after which the lens is discarded and replaced. Peroxide-, preservative-, or alcohol-based care products can be used with frequent replacement lenses.

Disposable lenses have a life span of one day up to one or two weeks, after which the lens is discarded and replaced. Clinical preferences for disposable lens favor preservative- or alcohol-based care products versus peroxide products. In contrast, durable hydrogel lenses should be care for by using peroxide products (see Chapter 8).

Daily wear implies that a lens can be worn throughout the day but must be removed prior to sleeping. It must also be cleansed and disinfected by a specified care product system. An extended wear lens can be worn throughout the day and night for a maximum of 7 days without lens removal. When this lens is removed, it must be discarded or disinfected for re-use. Flexible wear allows a patient to wear a lens mainly on a daily wear schedule. However, when necessary, the patient can sleep with the lens still inserted (ie, during travel, outdoor activities, etc.). Flexible wear is considered a clinical compromise and an optimal fit for most patients who have variable wear schedules.

All extended wear materials can be worn as daily or flexible wear. However, not all daily wear lenses can be worn as flexible or extended wear unless the Food and Drug Administration (FDA) approves them for that purpose.

Classification by Chemistry

Hydrogel material (or "water gelatin-plastic") is the primary material used in soft contact lenses. This material is classified as hydrophilic or "water-loving." Lens makers use a simple monomer as the building block for the polymer. There are several monomers that are traditionally used in the chemistry of hydrogel lenses. HEMA (2-hydroxyethylmethacrylate) is the original and most widely used. Other agents used in hydrogel materials are shown in Table 4-2.

Table 4-1.
Classification of Hydrogel Lenses According to Wear and Replacement Schedule

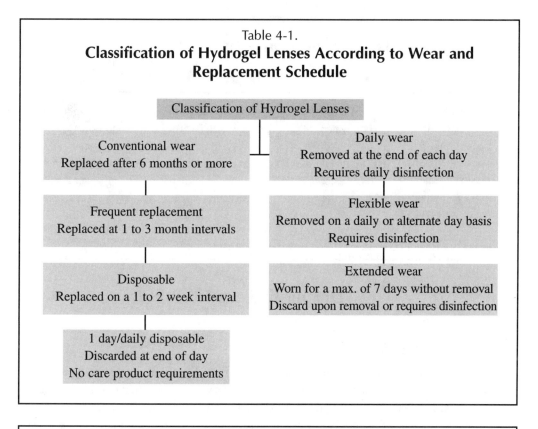

Classification of Hydrogel Lenses

Conventional wear
Replaced after 6 months or more

Daily wear
Removed at the end of each day
Requires daily disinfection

Frequent replacement
Replaced at 1 to 3 month intervals

Flexible wear
Removed on a daily or alternate day basis
Requires disinfection

Disposable
Replaced on a 1 to 2 week interval

Extended wear
Worn for a max. of 7 days without removal
Discard upon removal or requires disinfection

1 day/daily disposable
Discarded at end of day
No care product requirements

Table 4-2.
Hydrogel Polymers

EGDMA (ethylene glycol dimethacrylate)	Increases polymer stability
Methacrylic acid (MA)	Increases water content
Methyl Methacrylate (MMA)	Additional strength
Vinyl pyrrolidine (VP)	Increases the water content
Styrene	Increases the refractive index
Divinylbenzene	Increases stability

Hydrogel lens are classified by two characteristics: ionic character and water content. The ionic character of a lens is based on polymerization. Polymerization occurs by using either photochemical (ultraviolet) curing or a thermochemical (heat) process. These processes establish the final refractive index, water content, stability, and ionic character of the lens.[1] The lenses are then categorized by the FDA based on their chemistry (Table 4-3). The ionic character (ionic or nonionic) of the material is associated with the depositing nature of the lens.

The water content is physical property of the material which is classified as low to moderate (50% or less) or high (50% or higher). The classification of daily versus extended wear is based on the FDA stipulations pertaining to the oxygen requirements of the cornea in order to prevent swelling.

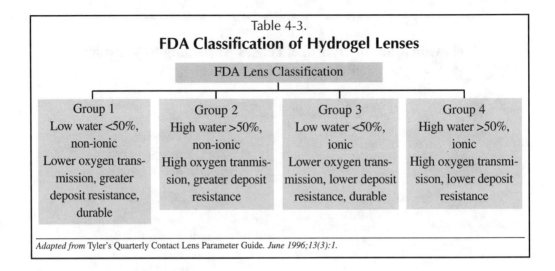

Table 4-3.
FDA Classification of Hydrogel Lenses

FDA Lens Classification			
Group 1	Group 2	Group 3	Group 4
Low water <50%, non-ionic	High water >50%, non-ionic	Low water <50%, ionic	High water >50%, ionic
Lower oxygen transmission, greater deposit resistance, durable	High oxygen tranmission, greater deposit resistance	Lower oxygen transmission, lower deposit resistance, durable	High oxygen transmission, lower deposit resistance

Adapted from Tyler's Quarterly Contact Lens Parameter Guide. *June 1996;13(3):1.*

Diagnostic Lens Fit

Lens Type Selection

The selection of a lens is based on patient education regarding the available lens types and /or patient's lens needs based on a detailed interview. The interview should elicit information regarding the patient's preference towards daily, flexible, or extended wear. The interviewer should determine if the patient would prefer disposable, frequent replacement, or durable lenses, as well ask if the individual desires a cosmetic change to eye color. Finally, questions pertaining to occupation and avocation are required to determine limitations on contact lens wear that may require safety eyewear or more frequently replaced lenses. The combination of objective clinical data and subjective input from the patient will allow the fitter to determine the best diagnostic or trial lens.

Tables 4-4 and 4-5 address lens advantages and disadvantages.

Base Curve Selection

The BC of the lens is traditionally based on the keratometric values of the central corneal curvature. However, keratometry should not be relied on for the sole determination of the BC selection. A diagnostic lens is required to assure the proper fit. Hydrophilic lens BCs range from 8.0 to 9.2 mm. The majority of fits will be successful between 8.5 and 8.8 mm.[2] In order to determine the initial BC, central flat keratometry can be used. Simply add a "swell factor" of approximately 1.3 mm to 1.4 mm (as discussed in Chapter 2) to the flat keratometric value.

Power Selection

Lens power selection is based on the manifest refraction with vertex correction (see chart in Appendix). Soft lenses, due to their inherent lack of "shape," will drape and conform to the contour of the cornea. Hydrogel lenses, unlike rigid gas permeable lenses, will not be correct for astigmatism unless specifically designed to do so (see Chapter 6). A spherical soft lens can "mask" a small amount of astigmatism, however. This is done by using the spherical equivalent

Table 4-4.
Comparison of Hydrogel Lens Types

Category	Durable Lenses	Frequent Replacement	Disposable Lenses
Cost to patient	3	2 to 3	2 to 3
Profit to the practice	1 to 2	2 to 3	2 to 3
Handling characteristics	3 to 4	2 to 3	2 to 3
Adverse reactions/complications	2 to 3	1 to 2	1
Related care product: ease of use	3 to 4	2 to 3	1 to 2
Related care product: compliance	1	2 to 3	3 to 4
Related care product: cost to patient	3 to 4	2 to 3	1 to 2

1 = low, poor   2 = low to average, average   3 = average to high, good   4 = high, excellent

Table 4-5.
Comparison of Hydrogel Wearing Schedules

Category	Daily Wear	Flexible Wear	Extended Wear
Cost to patient	2 to 3	2 to 3	3 to 4
Profit to the practice	2 to 3	2 to 3	3
Handling characteristics	3 to 4	2 to 3	1 to 2
Adverse reactions/complications	1 to 2	2 to 3	4
Related care product: ease of use	2 to 3	2 to 3	None required
Related care product: compliance	2 to 3	2	None required
Related care product: cost to patient	3	2	None required

1 = low, poor   2 = low to average, average   3 = average to high, good   4 = high, excellent

of the patient's refractometric measurement. The spherical equivalent is calculated as half the cylinder added to the sphere power. For example: -2.00 − 1.00 x 180 has a spherical equivalent of -2.50 (ie, half of -1.00 is -0.50; -0.50 added to -2.00 = -2.50).

The diagnostic lens power is based on the effective power. This is defined as the adjustment in lens power from spectacle plane to corneal plane. If a lens is moved into a closer proximity to the cornea, the power must be increased by adding plus. This will allow the image to remain focused on the fovea. If power is not increased, the image would be displaced beyond the fovea, leaving the patient undercorrected. If the lens is moved away from the cornea, the power needs to be reduced to diverge light and maintain the position of the foveal image. An acronym for this effect is CAP—Closer Add Plus. Effectivity becomes appreciable in calculations at powers greater than ±4.00 diopters.

Power effectivity, as it pertains to soft contact lenses, is dramatically different versus rigid lenses. Since a rigid lens maintains its shape, it is assumed there will always be a tear layer effect requiring power compensation in each meridian. However, with soft or hydrogel lenses, the tear layer is negated due to the lack of lens rigidity and the material's ability to contour to the corneal surface. The tear layer which does exist is minute and demonstrates no power effect.

Formula for Effectivity

$$F_E = F_a / (1 - dF_a)$$

F_E = effective power (in diopters)   d = measured vertex distance (in millimeters)

F_a = spectacle lens power (in diopters)

Placement of the Lens on the Eye

On the initial fitting of the hydrogel contact lens, the fitter must place the lens on the patient's eye. Explain to the patient that the lens is like a piece of plastic wrap that will fit the contour of the eye. It will first feel as if an eyelash is in the eye, but will be unnoticeable in a few minutes. Persistent foreign body sensation implies a poor fit (flat), or an inverted or defective lens.

Most patients will be highly motivated at the first visit, although some may be anxious enough to cause a fainting response. As a precaution, it is best to slightly recline the examining chair with the patient's head laid back against the headrest when inserting a lens for the first time. Ammonia salts should also be kept handy.

To place the lens on the patient's eye, use the following procedure:

1) Wash your hands in front of the patient (this acts as reinforcement).

2) Recline the chair and place the patient's head against the headrest.

3) Explain what you are going to do.

4) Grasp the upper lid margin with your index finger by placing an open hand on the patient's forehead, with your thumb on the temporal aspect of the patient's head. (This creates support and allows the fitter to have some control of the patient's head.)

5) Put the lens on your index finger. Place your thumb on the patient's cheek and grasp the lower lid margin with your middle finger.

6) Ask to patient to look away from you and place the lens onto the temporal aspect of the eye. Avoid touching the lens to the patient's eyelashes, which would cause reflex blinking. (By having the patient look away and introducing the lens from the periphery, the patient will not be aware of the lens coming onto the eye.)

7) After the lens has been placed onto the eye, continue holding the lids apart and have the patient slowly look into the lens. The cornea will slide underneath the lens.

8) Continue to hold the lids and have the patient slowly look about. Look for air pockets underneath the lens surface. (If air pockets exist and the lid is closed quickly, the lens will buckle and dislodge.)

9) Release the lids slowly and have the patient close the eye. Gently massage the upper lid to force out any air pockets.

10) Repeat with the next lens.

Lens removal should be easier and quicker. Follow the same procedures as above to secure the eyelids (steps 1 through 5). Then:

6) Have the patient look upward. Place your index finger on the 6 o'clock position of the contact lens and slide it down slightly. This will break the surface tension between the lens and the cornea.

7) While holding the lens in place with your index finger, quickly and lightly squeeze or pinch the lens between your thumb and index finger to grab the lens from the eye.

Evaluating the Fit

An efficient diagnostic lens fitting method will expedite the process and decrease chair time at aftercare visits (Table 4-6). There are two methods of diagnostic lens fits: a bilateral same lens and a bilateral comparative lens fit. The "same lens" diagnostic fit is used in the majority of cases where there is clinical confidence in the lens design to complement the visual, comfort, and physiological needs of the patient. In this case, the same lens (ie, same lens type and parameters) is placed on both eyes.

In the bilateral comparative method a different lens design is placed on each eye and compared. The examiner should ask the patient which lens feels better on the eye (physical comfort, not visual). If one lens feels significantly better, or if there is less lens awareness of one versus the other, it suggests that the lens with lesser awareness is probably tighter. In contrast, an *excessive* amount of lens awareness would imply that the lens is fit more loosely (ie, flatter). In either case, it will tell the fitter what to expect with slit lamp examination.

With either method, the lens should be observed immediately upon insertion in order to monitor its initial "on eye" fitting characteristics. The lens should then be allowed to settle on the eye, then observed again. (Examiners vary in their opinion as to how long the lens should be allowed to settle, from 2 to 30 minutes. This author prefers an immediate lens evaluation on lens insertion and once again after a 5-minute settlement time.) During the time of equilibration, the lens will start to dehydrate and grow steeper on the eye.[3, 4, 5, 6, 7, 8, 9, 10]

Lens Coverage

The lens diameter should extend far enough beyond the limbus to allow for proper draping over the conjunctiva. There should be a minimum of 1.0 mm limbal-to-lens-edge clearance in order to avoid corneal exposure during blinking. If corneal exposure occurs during the blink, the patient will have an increased foreign body sensation and may exhibit minor punctate staining. Hydrophilic lens diameters range from 12.5 to 16 mm, averaging between 13.8 to 14.5 mm.

Lens Centration

Lens centration defines the position of the hydrogel lens in relation to the corneal diameter (Figure 4-1). Optimal centration implies that there is equal lens material surrounding the cornea from limbus to lens edge. Lens centration can be measured by using an ocular reticule or a beam reticule (Figure 4-2). (An ocular reticule is a slit lamp eyepiece with an imprinted protractor and millimeter rule. It measures on a 0.3 mm scale at 10x and a 0.1 mm scale at 30x. The beam reticule can be calibrated against a measuring rule and will not vary with a change in magnification.) An optimal centration is 0.8 to 1.2 mm.

Lens Movement

Primary gaze lens movement is considered the most sensitive indicator of lens movement when compared to lateral and upward gaze measures. Primary gaze movement is measured after the lens has settled following the blink. Once settled, ask the patient to blink normally (without excessive force), and watch the translation. Up-gaze movement is measured in the same manner as the patient gazes slightly upward. (This measure depends on the patient's ocular position in up-gaze. The higher the up-gaze, the greater the lid interaction.) Lid and lens interaction will increase the amount of translation due to the increased force associated with lid tension.

To measure lens movement in primary gaze, narrow the slit lamp beam so that it fits between the limbus and the lens edge, making a note of the beam width. Have the patient blink, and measure the vertical movement of the lens through the beam width. Movement is acceptable if it is 50% of the beam, or 0.4 to 0.5 mm.

Table 4-6.
Fitting Characteristics of Disposable Hydrogel Contact Lenses

Characteristic/Measure	Flat	Optimal	Steep
Primary gaze	0.51mm >	0.15 to 0.50 mm	< 0.14 mm
Up-gaze	0.65 mm >	0.45 to .60 mm	< 0.4 mm
Lateral gaze	0.65 mm >	0.45 to 0.60 mm	< 0.4 mm
Tightness percentage (subj.)	< 40%	45% to 55%	60% >
Tear reservoir = edge accumulation with macromolecular NaFl (0 to 4 scale)	0 to 1	2 to 3	4
Vessel impingement = Compression of lens edge onto superficial conj. vessels	0 to 1 *No vessel dilation or constriction to either side of lens edge, no conj. drag on blink*	2 to 3 *Minimal vessel dilation or constriction to either side of lens edge, minor conj. drag on blink*	4 *Vessel dilation to external peripheral lens edge with associated constriction to the internal periphery of lens edge with significant. conj. drag on blink*
Lens decentration (estim.) Limbus to lens edge Avg. corneal diameter = 12 mm	14 mm lens diameter vs. 14.5 mm lens diameter (LD-VID) ± PGM/2* (averaged decentration)	(optimal centration)	(averaged decentration)
Superior	1.17 to 1.42 mm	1 to 1.25 mm	0.93 to 1.15 mm
Inferior	0.83 to 1.02 mm	1 to 1.25 mm	1.07 to 1.32 mm
Nasal	0.83 to 1.02 mm	1 to 1.25 mm	1.07 to 1.32 mm
Temporal	1.17 to 1.42 mm	1 to 1.25 mm	0.93 to 1.15 mm
Edge fluting	Yes (inf. nasal)	None	None
Coverage	Potential corneal exposure inf. nasal	Complete	Potential corneal exposure superior temporal
Additional characteristics to be evaluated	Lid tension (0 to 4)	Tear meniscus (0 to 0.4)	Iris diameter
Evaluation of fit	Optimal: A fit which demonstrates proper movement, centration, physiological and physical comfort, and visual quality. On lens movement there is complete coverage of the cornea without limbal exposure.	Marginal : A fit which demonstrates proper movement, centration, physiological and physical comfort, and visual quality. Movement may allow the lens to come into close proximity of the limbus but still maintains complete coverage of the cornea without limbal exposure.	Unacceptable: A fit which demonstrates improper movement; poor centration; potentially decreases physiological or physical comfort, and visual quality. Movement allows the lens to translate onto the corneal surface or forbids translation due to tightness.

*LD = lens diameter, VID = visible iris diameter, PGM = primary gaze movement

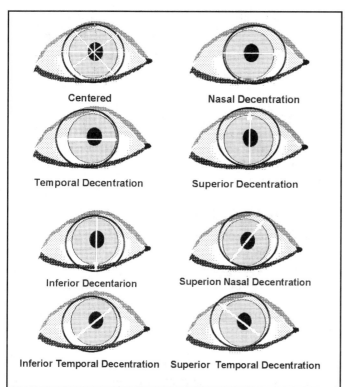

Figure 4-1. Lens decentration.

Centered   Nasal Decentration

Temporal Decentration   Superior Decentration

Inferior Decentarion   Superion Nasal Decentration

Inferior Temporal Decentration   Superior Temporal Decentration

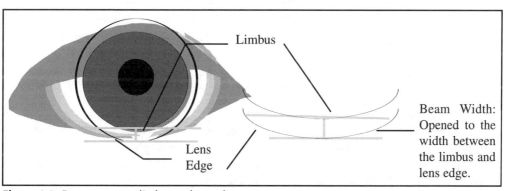

Figure 4-2. Beam measure limbus to lens edge.

Lateral movement is the least reliable of the three measures. The patient is asked to first look forward into primary gaze, then to look left, center, then right. The amount of movement is approximated based on the amount of lens lag (ie, the amount of lens that doesn't 'keep up' with the cornea when the eye is moved).

The Push-Up test is used to differentiate lid interaction from other lens movement influences. It is considered the most reliable test for determining the adequacy of the hydrogel lens fit. Lens tightness is evaluated by pushing the lower lid against the lens edge and grading the freedom of lens movement. A grade of 50% indicates optimal lens tightness. In contrast, a grade of 100% indicates no movement and 0% indicates a lens that is not maintained on the cornea. The normal range is between 40% (less restriction of movement) and 60% (greater restriction of movement). Forty percent easily moves upward due to less resistance but recovers slowly due to increased lid interaction.

Fifty percent moves upward easily and recovers with equal quickness. Sixty percent is difficult to move upward but recovers very quickly due to the steepness of the cornea/lens relationship.

Durable (conventional) lenses will generally have greater lens movement in all gazes.

Other Fitting Notes

Peripheral fitting relationships should be observed and documented at various intervals on the initial lens fit. When a lens is first placed onto the eye, the edge may lift away from the conjunctival surface. This implies that the lens is either inverted or excessively flat. If the lens is flat, it may bulk and create a funnel-like appearance called *edge fluting* (Figure 4-3). If the lens is tight, the edge will bear or compress onto the perilimbal conjunctival vessels and cause vascular dilatation peripheral to the lens edge.

Finally, the overall lens fit can be rated as acceptable if there is complete corneal coverage with an optimal range of lens movement (as demonstrated by the Push-Up test and primary gaze movement). The fit is unacceptable if there is any excessive movement, with corneal exposure on the blink. The lens can be judged as a marginally acceptable fit if there is a normal range of movement and appreciable lens decentration close to the limbus (within 0.1 to 0.2 mm) without exhibiting corneal exposure.

Over-Refractometry

After lens equilibration, visual acuity and a spherocylindrical over-refraction (SCO) should be performed.[11] The SCO is performed while the patient views his or her best line of achievable visual acuity. If necessary, introduce cylinder to determine if there is an appreciable difference in acuity. If there is an appreciable improvement in vision with added cylinder, a toric contact lens may be considered, or a cylinder-only spectacle overcorrection can be prescribed.

Patient Instructions and Aftercare

Note: See also Chapter 7.

Patient insertion and removal training should take place in a private and individualized session. Initial videotape education is quite beneficial in the training process. The tape should address the general questions posed by the majority of patients. Following video education, the trainer should discuss any additional questions and then proceed with insertion and removal (I & R) training. If a patient has had previous contact lens experience but has not worn lenses for some time, re-training is highly recommended. Never assume a patient is able to insert and remove a lens until he or she can prove it.

Aftercare schedules vary based on the type of lens being dispensed and the patient's previous experience with contact lenses. If a patient is wearing lenses for the first time, an initial lens wear schedule should be approximately 4 hours on the first and second day followed by an increase of 1 hour per day to a maximum of 8 hours. At this point, the patient should return to the office 1 week after the initial training session.

If the patient is interested in pursuing overnight lens wear, the previous schedule should be followed with the patient wearing the lens overnight 1 night prior to the 1 week visit. (This should only be done if the patient has not observed any adverse reactions prior to overnight lens use.) The 1 week progress check should be scheduled as close to the patient's waking hour as possible so the practitioner can look for signs of edema (such as straie and folds).

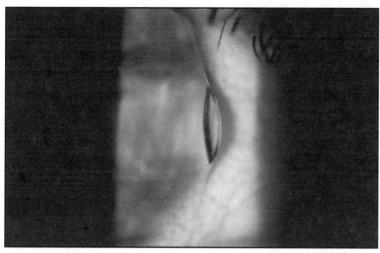

Figure 4-3. Edge fluting.

During the initial aftercare visit, patients should be questioned about their comfort level with I & R. They should be asked to demonstrate the proper method of lens care. At the same time, patients may be surveyed on general handling characteristics including the ability to see the lens in its storage case, determination of inversion, ease of insertion, ease of removal, physical comfort, visual quality, sense of lens durability, subjective level of acuity, requirement for and effect of wetting drops, and ocular redness.

Subjective lens evaluations are at times more essential in determining the best-fit scenario for a patient, rather than objective clinical measures. Difficulty in lens insertion and identifying an inverted lens are items that may frustrate the patient enough to discontinue lens use. These difficulties can easily be addressed with re-training or a new lens selection. It is vitally important to be aware of these concerns in order to optimize the contact lens fit.

References

1. Su KC. Chemistry of soft contact lens materials. In: Bennett E, Weissman BA, eds. *Clinical Contact Lens Practice.* Philadelphia, Pa: JB Lippincott Company: 1991.

2. Young G. Ocular sagittal height and soft contact lens fit. *Journal of the British Contact Lens Association.* 1992;15(4):45-48.

3. Pritchard N, Fonn D. Dehydration, lens movement, and dryness ratings of hydrogel contact lenses. *Ophthalmic Physiology.* July 1995;15(4):281-286.

4. Weschler S, et al. In vivo hydration of gel lenses. *International Contact Lens Clinic.* May/June 1983;5:154-157.

5. Andrasko G, Schoessler JP. The effect of humidity on the dehydration of soft contact lens on the eye. *International Contact Lens Clinic.* September/October 1980;9:30-32.

6. Andrasko G. The amount and time course of soft contact lens dehydraton. *Contact Lens Forum.* May/June 1982;53(3):207.

7. Andrasko G. Hydrogel dehydration in various environments. *International Contact Lens Clinic.* January/February 1983;10(1):22-27.

8. Brennan NA, et al. Hydrogel lens dehydration: material-dependent phenomenon? *Contact Lens Forum.* April 1987;28-29.

9. Brennan NA, Efron N, Bruce AS, Duldig DI, Russo NJ. Dehydration of hydrogel lenses: environmental influences during normal wear. *American Journal of Optometry and Physiological Optics.* 1988;65(4):277-281.

10. Brennan NA, Lowe R, Efron N, Harris MG. In vivo dehydration of disposable (AcuVue) contact lenses. *Optom Vis Sci.* 1990;67(3):201-203.

11. Daniels KD. Evaluating a new molded disposable lens. *Contact Lens Spectrum.* December 1995;12:42-46.

Chapter 5

Rigid Gas Permeable Design

KEY POINTS

- The basic rule of lens design: create a complementary relationship between the anterior surface of the cornea and the back surface of the contact lens.

- There should be an even distribution of the lens mass over the paracentral (3 to 4 mm) corneal area.

- The BC is designed to conform to the corneal cap, establishing an alignment.

- Any residual lacrimal lens effect will manifest in either a plus or minus and/or toric over-refraction. The over-refraction can either be incorporated into the contact lens power or minimized by flattening the BC and/or decreasing the OZD.

- A bearing ("negative tear layer") effect of the lens onto the corneal surface will create pressure on the corneal cap while forcing tear fluids to the periphery of the lens.

- Alignment ("plano tear layer") is a method of designing the BC and OZD in order to support the lens evenly across the corneal cap without bearing.

- Clearance ("positive tear layer") implies that the lens is fit steep, when compared to the curvature of the central cornea.

Design Concepts

There are several types of rigid lens designs that can be made based on the shape and contours of the cornea (Figure 5-1). The two basic corneal shapes are spherical and aspherical (toric). Spherical implies that the cornea has minimal topographic variation, described as a low e (eccentricity) value. Aspheric implies that the corneal surface is comprised of a series of sections with progressive power and curvature changes. Toric implies that a separate sphere or ellipse is fit to each power meridian of the cornea.

Spherical and toric designs are derived from basic keratometry measures. Simply, the rigid lens is designed to match the spherical or toric geometry of the cornea. In contrast, an aspheric design assumes that the cornea will be steeper centrally and will then flatten to the periphery in a non-spherical progression.

The goal of rigid lens design is to create a complementary relationship between the anterior surface of the cornea and the back surface of the contact lens. To achieve this relationship, several basic rules should be applied:

1) The lens should smoothly align and contour the apical and mid-peripheral regions of the cornea. This area includes the corneal cap and the mid-periphery to approximately 10 to 11 mm.

2) The lens should exhibit trace clearance or trace bearing or touch over the corneal cap. (Touch and bearing are similar phrases differentiated by the apparent degree or lack of lens alignment. Touch implies that the lens presses on the cornea allowing for a trace to 1-sodium fluorescein pattern versus bearing, which implies a much greater pressing of the lens on the cornea allowing for a 1⁻ to 2⁻ sodium fluorescein. The 'minus' implies a lack of NaFl.)

3) The design should achieve an even alignment surrounding the pupil, encompassing the paracentral 3 to 4 mm.

4) An alignment to the paracentral or mid-peripheral area is critical in order to properly support the lens on the corneal cap. The lens should have an even distribution of mass over the cornea.

5) The lens should maintain adequate movement without obstruction.

6) A proper lens design should avoid naso-temporal decentration or rocking. If rocking occurs, the lens will induce epithelial chafing with secondary 3-9 staining.

Additionally, rigid lens design and fitting scenarios will abide by several basic rules. (These are not steadfast, but are good guidelines to problem solving and to a highly successful fit rate with optimal comfort, vision, and long-term health.)

1) The lens will always seek the steepest part of the cornea.

2) The lens will move along the path of least mechanical obstruction or in the flattest fitting meridian.

3) A steep lens will move towards the corneal apex while a flat lens will move to the flatter periphery.

4) The lens will tend to be tighter in the mid-periphery.

5) The lens will tend to seek the largest area of bearing/alignment, thereby establishing an equilibrated support of lens mass and pressure over the corneal surface.

6) A flat-fitting lens is more influenced by lid interaction, while a steep fit is influenced by central corneal contours.

7) The basic principles of SAM (steeper add minus)/FAP (flatter add plus)/CAP (closer add plus) should be applied when prescribing lens power. A general rule is as follows: A 0.05 diopter change in curvature is equivalent to a 0.25 change in millimeters.

8) Lid interaction has a major influence on the lens fit and position, but is not predicted in topography.

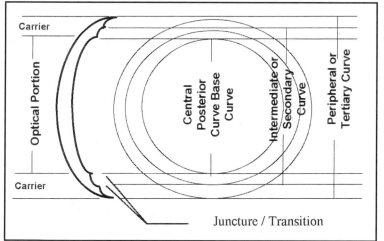

Figure 5-1. Lens design parameters and fitting characteristics.

Hard and Rigid Lens Materials and Parameters

There are several basic materials available for hard and rigid lens design.

PMMA is referred to as a "hard lens material." Even though it is a very stable and long-lasting material, it is has an extremely poor oxygen transmission capability. SA (silicone acrylate), followed by FSA (fluorinated silicone acrylate), allows for increased oxygen transmissibility. These two materials are sometimes referred to as "semi-soft" or "semi-hard." SA and FSA polymers facilitate more oxygenated tear and gas exchange, reducing lens-induced edema and corneal distortions, while increasing the patient's comfort and wearing time.

The Dk or Diffusion Coefficient value is the oxygen transmissibility or permeability of a material. The Dk can be expressed in relation to the center thickness (L) of the material by the equation Dk/L. This defines the ability of oxygen to transport across a material of known thickness. This value is directly related to the EOP. A higher Dk value will exhibit a lower incidence of corneal edema, particularly under extended wear conditions.[1]

Fluorine has become a primary additive to rigid lens polymer chemistry. Fluorine has no affinity to oxygen, thereby increasing the material's Dk value. Fluorine has a greater level of flexibility, decreasing potential lens warping. However, fluorine does decrease the hardness of the material, making it easier to scratch or crack. Still, fluorinated silioacrylate materials have become the favored material of rigid lens fitters.

Base Curve and Fitting Relationships

The BC, or CPC, is the primary curve of the lens. It is designed to contour the anterior corneal surface and tear film. The BC is designed to approximate a near alignment to the cornea in order to decrease or avoid the lacrimal lens effect and compensate for any corneal cylinder.

The BC's relationship to the cornea may be referred to as bearing, alignment, or clearance. Bearing suggests that the lens is fitting flat on the cornea, forcing the tear film to the periphery. Alignment suggests that the tear film and lens mass are evenly distributed on the corneal surface. Clearance implies that the lens is steeper than the keratometric value, exhibiting an increased tear film layer in the central portion of the lens (ie, the lens "clears" the corneal cap).

The BC of the lens is selected based on either keratometric measures (K's) or topography. The lens is generally fit "on K," flatter than K, or steeper than K.

An "on K" (alignment) fit implies that the curvature is equal to the flattest keratometric reading. This type of fit allows a trace clearance without bearing, yet maintains sufficient lid interaction (Figure 5-2). An alignment fit diminishes, but does not negate, the lacrimal lens or tear film effect. Thus, this method is appropriate for low cylindrical power correction. An alignment fit encourages proper tear fluid exchange.

A "flatter than flat K" fit involves using a BC flatter than the flattest meridian of the cornea. It will exhibit a bearing effect on the corneal cap, allowing for increased lid interaction. This is also called a lid attachment or a superior aperture fit (Figure 5-3). Bearing may cause a minus lens effect, requiring a plus power compensation (FAP-flatter add plus).

In a "steeper than flat K" fit, the curve has a dioptric value slightly steeper than the flattest meridian of the cornea. This will allow for central clearance of the lens. In this scenario, the lens will position itself centrally on the cornea. Such a fit is also called a palpebral aperture fit or a slightly inferior fit (Figure 5-4).

It is important to note that any residual lacrimal lens or tear film effect will manifest in a plus or minus and/or toric over-refraction. The over-refraction can either be incorporated into the lens power or minimized by flattening the BC and/or decreasing the OZD. The latter two modifications will align or bear the lens onto the corneal cap, virtually eliminating the lacrimal lens effect.

The BC selection should be biased to the amount of CA. If there is a low corneal cylinder power, a "flatter than flat K" or "on K" curve is selected. The goal of an "on K" fit is to align the back surface of the contact to the cornea and negate the corneal cylinder/lacrimal lens effect.

The OZD, more so than the overall lens diameter, will have a direct proportional effect on the alignment of the lens to the cornea. Larger diameters mimic a steeper lens effect while a smaller diameter mimics a flatter lens effect. Larger OZDs will yield a subtle increase in central clearance or a plus tear lens effect, thereby requiring a minus power compensation (SAM-steeper add minus).

Lens Diameter Determination

The lens diameter may be selected using the following guidelines:

1) The lens diameter should allow the superior lid to support the upper portion of the lens at all times.

2) The lens diameter should be appropriate to the palpebral aperture width. A smaller width requires a smaller lens and vice versa.

3) The lens diameter should be approximately 2.0 to 2.5 mm smaller than the visible iris diameter, or 1.2 to 1.5 mm from the limbus to the lens edge (Figure 5-5).

4) A larger lens diameter requires a more complex PCR system or an aspheric PCR.

The BC selection should be biased to the amount of CA. If there is a low corneal cylinder power, a "flatter than flat K" or "on K" curve is selected. The goal of an "on K" fit is to align the back surface of the contact lens to the cornea and negate the corneal cylinder/lacrimal lens effect. As noted in Table 5-1, the OZD and the overall lens diameter will have a marked effect on the fitting characteristic of a rigid lens.

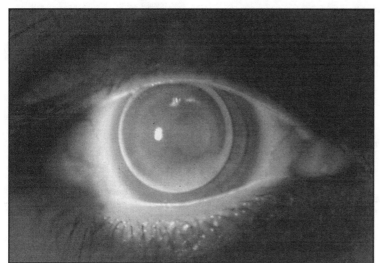

Figure 5-2. Alignment fit.

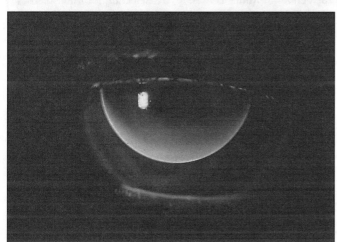

Figure 5-3. Superior aperture/lid attachment fit.

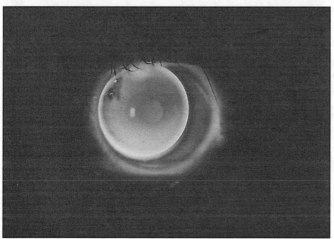

Figure 5-4. Palpebral aperture fit.

Figure 5-5. Limbus to lens edge clearance with rigid gas permeable lenses.

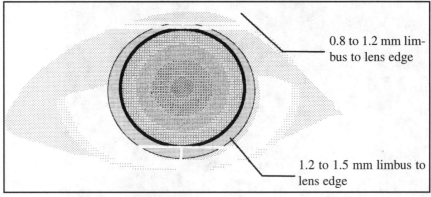

0.8 to 1.2 mm limbus to lens edge

1.2 to 1.5 mm limbus to lens edge

Table 5-1.
BC Selection Based on Corneal Cylinder

Corneal Cylinder	BC Selection for Minus Lenses: 9.2 Lens Diameter	BC Selection for Minus Lenses: 9.6 Lens Diameter
plano to -0.50 DC	0.50 D flatter	0.75 D flatter
0.75 DC to 1.25 DC	0.25 D flatter	0.50 D flatter
1.50 DC to 2.00 DC	On K	0.25 D flatter
2.25 DC to 2.75 DC	0.25 D steeper	On K
3.00 DC to 3.50 DC	0.50 D steeper	0.25 D steeper

For plus lenses, fit the BC 0.25 to 0.50 steeper than recommended for minus lenses.

Adapted from Morgan BW. RGP material selection and design. Eyequest. *1994;4:49-58.*

Lens Fitting Methods

Lid Attachment/Korb Design

The lid attachment, or superior aperture (sometimes called the Korb Fitting Philosophy) uses a unique edge contour in conjunction with the anterior and posterior curve system. This is done to encourage lid attachment. Lid attachment implies that the lens will translate vertically with lid and blink motion.[2] The Korb design varies the BC, PCR or contour, edge contour, ET, lens diameter, and lens mass to control the amount of lid attachment. The advantage of this type of fit is a reduction of epithelial drying due to anterior contouring and its thin edge design. Comfort is enhanced due to the thin lens edge and its ability to adhere to the lid during translation. The only disadvantage in this lens design is the potential for induced superior corneal bearing and molding.

Lid Interactive or Modified Korb Design

In the lid interactive (or modified Korb design), the BC and OZD relationship create an alignment fit rather than the bearing effect as seen with Korb or superior aperture/lid attachment fits. Lid interactive implies that the lens will assume a superior position on the cornea using the lid margin to brace the superior portion of the lens and allow it to move in concert with the lid.

There are several general rules for the BC, PCR, optic zone, and lens diameter design for lid interactive fits. These are as follows.

1) The BC selection will be slightly flatter than the flat keratometric value, premised by the amount of corneal cylinder.

2) The optic zone diameter (OZD) should be equal to or slightly greater than the base curve in millimeters. OZD = BCR + (0.1 mm to 0.3 mm). An OZD equal to the BC will reduce the restriction of lens movement.

3) PCRs are spherical curves which are flattened progressively in relation to the BC.

4) The overall lens diameter should be have a limbus-to-lens-edge clear zone of approximately 1.2 mm to 1.5 mm.

5) The optic zone should be approximately 0.5 mm to 1 mm larger than the pupil in dim illumination. (Patients with larger pupils may appreciate a prismatic effect from the juncture.)

Interpalpebral Lens Design or Central Palpebral Fit

Interpalpebral design (or central palpebral fitting) uses a steeper than the flat keratometric value and a smaller lens diameter. The lens is designed to fit between the superior and inferior lids while remaining centralized during and after the blink. Due to the steepness of the base curve, the lens will exhibit a significant clearance pattern. There are several basic rules to follow in designing an interpalpebral design.

1) The OZD is small in order to complement a steeper BC.

2) The OZD should be approximately 0.2 mm to 0.3 mm less than the millimeter value of the BC.

3) The BC will be one-third (0.33) to a one-fourth (0.25) "steeper than flat K."

4) The PCRs will be limited to a secondary and peripheral tricurve system due to a limited lens diameter.

5) Interpalpebral designs with low edge clearance will cause epithelial desiccation. This is relieved by using a smaller diameter with a higher edge lift.

Other Features

Aspheric or Hyperbolic PCRs

An aspheric or hyperbolic peripheral curves, specified by an e value, can be used in substitute for a specified PCR design. The use of an aspheric or hyperbolic curve is to reduce flare normally created by distinct junctures. When using a hyperbolic peripheral curve, it is best to design the base curve of the lens 0.25 mm flatter than normal in order to increase the peripheral clearance of the lens.

Design and Visual Effects of Junctures

If using a specifically designed PCR, juncture smoothness needs to be specified. The juncture is the meeting point between two curves. It has a shape similar to that of a prism. The patient will describe a poor juncture design via subjective compliants of poor comfort and/or the awareness of "halos or flare". They will often remark that "I can see the edge of the lens" or "lights appear to have a halo or elongation." The less blended the juncture, the more pronounced the effect. The juncture can be sharp to smooth as defined by the designer. The blend is specified as smooth, moderate, or heavy. If the juncture remains unblended, the lens will create excessive corneal desiccation, while increasing the patient's lens awareness and discomfort.

CT and Lens Mass

Rigid lens materials are usually slightly thicker than PMMA lenses due to the increased oxygen transmissibility and need to avoid lens flexure. CT recommendations for lens powers plano to -1.00 diopter are 0.17 mm to 0.20 mm followed by a decrease in thickness by 0.01 mm for each increase in diopter. CT should be increased by 0.02 mm for each diopter of CA.

Lenticulation

Lenticulation is a modification to the outer one-quarter of the lens. It is used to reduce the lens mass, allow for peripheral lens contouring with the upper lid, improve lens centration, and add structural strength to the lens. Lenticulation is incorporated when lens powers exceed ±4.00 diopters. It is at these powers that the periphery of the lens will either become excessively thin, as with plus lenses; or excessively thick, as with minus lenses. These lens designs may also be referred to as myoflange or hyperflange.

Edge Design

The design of the lens edge needs to be tapered and rounded in order to enhance tear fluid exchange and avoid epithelial desiccation. The optimal lens edge design should be smooth, rounded, and tapered anteriorly away from the cornea. A sharp edge design will cause a more significant level of 3-9 staining with epithelial desiccation.

Handling Tints and Dots

Since the lenses are generally small and difficult to see, it is best to order lenses with handling tints. Handling tints, usually blue, are dyes incorporated into the polymer prior to fabrication. Handling tints are also available in some materials in green, gray, and ice blue. For additional lens handling ease, a black dot can be impregnated onto the surface of the lens to indicate if the lens is a right or left lens. The dot is traditionally placed on the right lens.

Fluorescein Patterns

NaFl is an organic compound that combines with the tear film and accumulates underneath the contact lens. The NaFl pattern is best visualized using a cobalt blue light and a wratten yellow filter. The NaFl will fluoresce yellow/green, allowing the fitter to determine areas where the lens clears or touches the cornea (Figure 5-6).

After the lens has settled and the patient achieves an adequate level of comfort without excessive tearing, the fitter can proceed with the lens evaluation. A gross view of the lens should be made without the slit lamp in order to assure proper placement of the lens on the cornea. Then instill NaFl for further examination with a hand-held Burton (black light) lamp or slit lamp. The fluorescein pattern is evaluated for the following lens/cornea relationship: (1) bearing (2) clearance or (3) alignment at the apex or mid-periphery. This assessment is made separately within optical zone region, the mid-periphery, and within the PCR system. NaFl inspection requires grading the amount of pooling or the lack thereof.

An "on flat K" (alignment) fit is visualized as a faint or subtle amount of NaFl between the back surface of the lens and the cornea (Figure 5-7). An optimal alignment pattern is exhibited as an even fluorescence between the posterior lens surface and the anterior cornea.

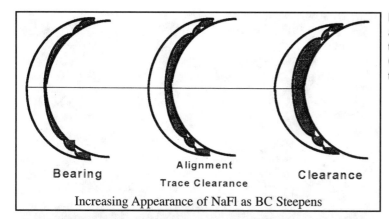

Figure 5-6. Fluorescein accumulation with "flatter than K" (bearing), "on K" (alignment), and "steeper than K" (clearance).

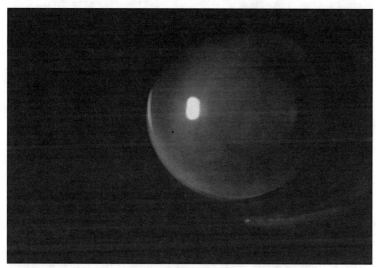

Figure 5-7. Alignment fit.

A flat or apical bearing fit will exhibit a darkened, hypo-fluorescent area centrally with increasing fluorescence peripherally (Figure 5-8). The bearing or touch effect of the lens will create pressure on the corneal cap while forcing tear fluids towards the periphery of the lens ("negative tear layer"). This is referred to as mid-peripheral clearance. The NaFl pattern is observed as a darkened central area or lack of visible NaFl under the lens at the central cornea, with increasing NaFl towards the periphery. Bearing of the contact lens can induce apical molding, which can result in a disk-shaped flattening of the cornea. In some cases, this is a desired scenario in order to re-shape the cornea.

A "steeper than K" fit implies that the lens is fit steep, when compared to the curvature of the central cornea. There will be increased central pooling of NaFl ("positive tear layer") because the contact vaults over the corneal surface (Figure 5-9). A steep or clearance pattern suggests stagnation of tear fluid and the entrapment of metabolic waste, sometimes seen as a "vortex" pattern of debris behind the lens (Figure 5-10).

An astigmatic pattern should demonstrate a subtle bearing along the flat meridian and a clearance along the steep meridian. This implies that with-the-rule cylinder (flat meridian at 180) should have bearing along axis 180 and clearance along axis 90 (Figure 5-11). In contrast, against-the-rule astigmatism (flat meridian at 90) will demonstrate a bearing along axis 90 and

Figure 5-8. Excessive central bearing/excessive peripheral clearance.

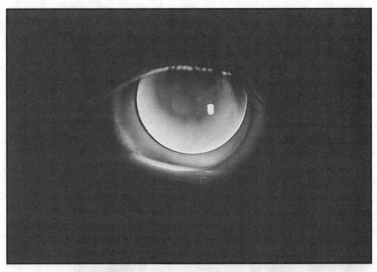

Figure 5-9. Excessive clearance/steep.

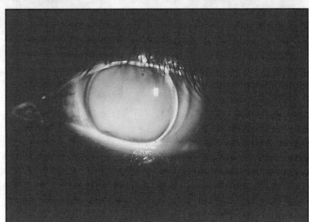

clearance along axis 180. These types of patterns are sometimes referred to as "figure-eight" or "dumbbell" (Figure 5-12).

OptT

Diagnostic and Aftercare Evaluations

The diagnostic fit and aftercare evaluations should be repeatable (Table 5-2). The examination should always start with visual acuity. The lens should be viewed grossly when inserted and then allowed to settle. This should be followed by a spherocylinder over-refraction. Judgment of centration, movement, and the NaFl pattern must be documented. Lens centration is graded based on its vertical and horizontal positioning on the cornea. Vertical positioning of the lens may be noted numerically as follows: 1 = superior, 2 = superior-central, 3 = central, 4 = central-inferior, or 5 = inferior. Horizontal positioning of the lens may be noted as 1 = nasal, 2 = temporal, 3 = central. Additionally, the lens/lid relation can be noted as lid attachment, partial lid attachment, or no lid attachment.

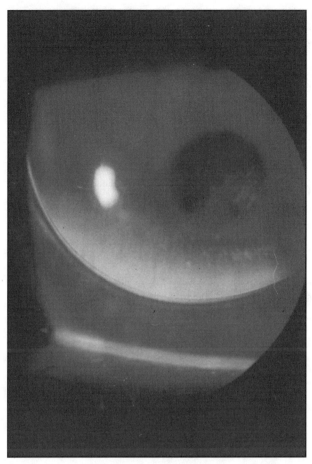

Figure 5-10. Inferior vortexing.

Troubleshooting Rigid Gas Permeable Fits

Many of the problems associated with rigid lenses are usually adaptive in nature. This is due to the patient's lack of familiarity with contact lenses and the variable comfort of the lens on the eye. Good education and preparation is critical to success. The patient must be prepared for the normal symptoms associated with rigid lenses. These include lens awareness, tearing, glare, photophobia, variable blink, and foreign body sensation. Over time, these will diminish to an unnoticeable level.

Lens Positioning

Correcting lens decentration requires thickness, curvature, and/or diameter adjustments.

If the NaFl pattern demonstrates bearing and the lens is decentered superiorly, a steeper BC or increase in the OZD should be considered (and vice versa for a lens that exhibits clearance).

Inferior decentration usually implies that the lens is steep or has excess mass. The lens should be re-ordered with a thin design, a flatter BC, smaller optic zone, and/or lenticulation (myoflange).

A nasal or temporal decentration is due to the movement of the lens along the path of least resistance, which is the flattest meridian. A with-the-rule lens fit has a flatter meridian at 180 that

Figure 5-11. Bearing and alignment relationships. Top: with-the-rule, bottom: against-the-rule. (Adapted from Caroline P, et al. Corneal topography and computerized contact lens fitting modules. *International Contact Lens Clinic.* 1994;21(5/6):185-195.)

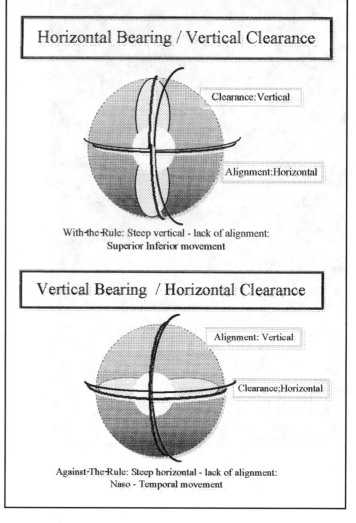

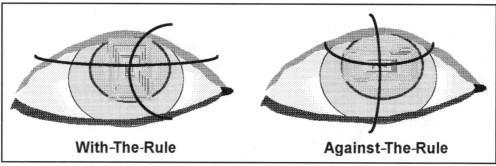

Figure 5-12. Astigmatic fluorescein pattern: with-the-rule "figure-eight" (left) and against-the-rule "dumbbell" (right).

Table 5-2.
Fitting Characteristics of Rigid Gas Permeable Contact Lenses

Characteristic/Measure

Overall NaFl: Optic zone of lens (central 7 to 8 mm)	Bearing: -2 (excessive flat) -1 (slightly flat < 10 µm)	Alignment = 0 10 to 20 µm	Clearance +1(slightly steep 20 to 40 µm) +2 (excessively steep 40 µm <)
Overall NaFl: Mid-periphery of lens (8 to 9.4 mm, 9.6 mm)	Bearing: -2 (excessive flat) -1 (slightly flat < 10 µm)	Alignment = 0 10 to 20 µm	Clearance +1 (slightly steep 20 to 40 µm) +2 (excessively steep 40 µm <)
Options: Documentation for NaFl relations	Bearing: -2 (excessive flat) -1 (slightly flat < 10 µm)	Alignment = 0 10-20 µm	Clearance +1 (slightly steep 20 to 40 µm) +2 (excessively steep 40 µm <)
Overall NaFl: PCR system of lens	-2 (extremely narrow < 0.1 µm) -1 (slightly narrow 0.10 to 0.20 µm)	Optimal = 0 0.20 to 0.30 µm	-2 extremely wide > 0.40 µm -1 slightly narrow 0.30 to 0.40 µm
Tear reservoir (microns) or axial edge clearance (AEC): accumulation of NaFl beneath the furthest extent of the lens edge	-2 insufficient < 40 µm -1 less than optimal ~60 µm	Optimal ~80 µm	+2 insufficient ~120 µm +1 less than optimal ~100 µm
Post blink position: Vertical	1 = Superior 2 = Superior/Central	3 = Central	4 = Central/Inferior 5 = Inferior
Post blink position: Horizontal	1 = Nasal	3 = Central	2 = Temporal
Lid relationship: related to vertical position	Complete lid attachment (noted as position 1)	Partial lid attachment (noted as position 2)	No lid interaction (noted as position 3, 4, or 5)
Pattern	With-the-rule	Against-the-rule	Oblique

Observable Patterns of   With-the-rule   Against-the-rule   Oblique
Astigmatism (area in gray (x 180)   (x 90)   (x 045)   (x 135)
implies clearance)

Clearance   Bearing
(steep meridian)   (Flat meridian)

Note: Micron (µm) measurements are estimated.

Table 5-2 continued.
Fitting Characteristics of Rigid Gas Permeable Contact Lenses
Documentation of Lens Position

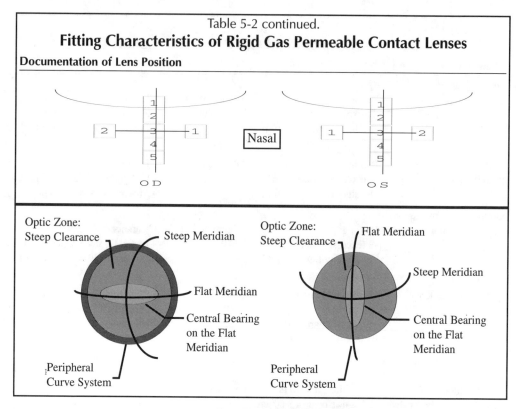

Optic Zone: Steep Clearance — Steep Meridian — Flat Meridian — Central Bearing on the Flat Meridian — Peripheral Curve System

Optic Zone: Steep Clearance — Flat Meridian — Steep Meridian — Central Bearing on the Flat Meridian — Peripheral Curve System

Figure 5-13. Lens pitch/paraffin.

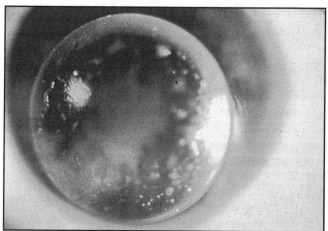

allows the lens to "rock" or decenter nasal and temporal. This rocking is evidenced as 3-9 corneal staining. To prevent horizontal decentration, increase resistance by increasing the OZD or incorporate a subtle steepening of the BC (subsequently flattening the PCR system).

Lens Flexure/Warping

Lens flexure is the ability of the lens to bend after each blink and then return to its original curvature. If lens flexure is excessive, the lens will warp. The patient may have fluctuating vision during lens wear and spectacle blur after removing the lenses.

To prevent flexure, materials should be selected which have enhanced dimensional stability. It is also beneficial to instruct patients to store lenses in solution to maintain BC profile.[3] Additionally, patients should be instructed to cleanse the lens in the palm of the hand using ample daily cleaner and not to clean the lens between the thumb and index finger. (The latter method tends to put pressure on the lens, inducing lens distortion.)

Residual Astigmatism

`OptT`

Residual astigmatism may be associated with lens flexure or uncorrected astigmatism. The lens should be verified for power and curvature. If a lens that was supposed to be spherical is found to have two power measures, it is either a toric design or the lens is warped. If the lens is spherical without distortion, the designer may assume that there is uncorrected astigmatism. In this case, a steeper BC, larger optic zone, or toric design should be considered.

Lens Clouding

`OptT`

Lens clouding means that the lens does not wet properly. A new lens that does not wet usually has residual manufacturer's pitch (wax) on the lens surface (Figure 5-13). Pitch can be removed with a solvent cleanser produced by the contact manufacturer. It is extremely important to re-clean the lens after using such a solvent, as well as to soak it in conditioning solution prior to dispensing. It is not advisable to polish the lens, because this will spread the pitch across the surface and make the situation worse.

Additional causes of lens clouding are the transfer of oils from hand creams, soaps, or cosmetics to the lens surface. Improper combination of care products and poor lens cleaning can also cause a non-wetting lens surface. To prevent or diminish the problem, instruct the patient on the proper use of care products, encourage frequent lens replacement (annual), and incorporate weekly enzymatic cleaning.

Spectacle Blur

Spectacle blur can be caused by corneal edema, lens over-wear, lens flexure, or lens-induced corneal molding. The patient will note vision changes throughout the day, as well as an inability to see clearly through spectacles. Additionally, he or she may complain of halos around lights and other glare problems. Corneal edema is associated with low Dk materials such as PMMA. To avoid corneal edema, the patient should be refit to a high Dk material with a slightly greater CT to prevent flexure. If the patient presents with corneal edema associated with low to moderate Dk materials, refit to a super-permeable material with a Dk value greater than 70. Frequent lens replacement should also be considered.

References

1. Benjamin WJ, et al. Hydrogel hypoxia: where we've been, where we're going. *Contact Lens Spectrum Supplemental.* September 1996;7.

2. Korb DR. et al. A new concept in contact lens design. Parts 1 and 2. *JAOA.* 1970;41(2):1023-1032.

3. Grohe RM. RGP problem solving. *Contact Lens Spectrum.* 1990;5:9.

Chapter 6

Astigmatic Lens Design

KEY POINTS

- Be conservative in toric correction; most patients can tolerate an astigmatic undercorrection with complete satisfaction.

- The lid will force a soft toric lens to rotate nasally on lid closure and temporally on opening.

- Transient blur implies that the soft toric lens may have a flat BC; this is easily remedied by using a steeper BC.

- Constant blurred vision with soft toric lenses implies that there is either an uncorrected refractive error or a constant misalignment of the lens axis.

- A back surface toric rigid lens is designed so that the posterior lens surface matches the cornea. It is used in cases where the cylinder induced by the lens equals the uncorrected subjective cylinder.

- Saddle fit rigid lenses are designed based on a full alignment to the two principle meridians of power.

- A low toric simulation rigid lens is fit "flatter than K" for the flat meridian, and undercorrects the steep meridian by approximately one-third.

- A bitoric lens design is analogous to designing a spherical lens for each meridian of the cornea with a fit factor that will flatten the BC in order to avoid the tear lens effect and compensate for residual astigmatism on the front surface of the lens.

Introduction

There are many considerations in astigmatic contact lens fitting. The proper lens should be selected based on material requirements and lens design, in conjunction with ocular health criteria and visual requirements. The decision process of fitting toric lenses (which correct for astigmatism by being more curved in one meridian than another) is fundamentally identical to soft and rigid lens fitting, except that there may be fewer lenses that meet the specified criteria developed during the decision process. There are several factors to be considered:

1) Is the cylindrical error strictly corneal in nature, or is there a lenticular component?
2) How does the corneal topography effect the fit?
3) What is the patient's visual sensitivity to the cylindrical error?
4) Which lens design and material will best suit the needs of the patient?

Definition of Astigmatism

Astigmatism is a non-pathological condition in which light entering the eye is not focused as a single point on the retina. This is due to variant curves of the cornea or a misalignment of the crystalline lens. The light that enters the eye is focused as two separate line foci at two distinct distances apart from each other due to the differences in the power meridians of the cornea or lens. The effect produced is a general blur at distance and near that may appear as a "double image." The clearest image that can be produced with best refractive correction is found at the midpoint between the two images (called the "circle of least confusion"). Cylinder, which has a defined power (plus or minus, at a specific axis or line of orientation), is used to correct astigmatism (Figure 6-1).

There are several types of astigmatism, including regular and irregular, residual, induced, and internal.

1) In regular astigmatism there is a 90 degree angle between each power meridian.

2) Irregular astigmatism has an angle between meridians which is not 90 degrees. It is usually associated with pathology.

3) Residual astigmatism is the difference between corneal and lenticular astigmatism, or the mathematical difference between corneal cylinder (as measured with the keratometer, for example) and the subjective refractive cylinder (as measured during refractometry).

4) Induced astigmatism is associated with contact lens-related flexure or with an acquired misalignment of the lens/cornea/tear relationship due to surgery or trauma.

Previous Lens Experience, Material and Design Selection

It is critical to understand the patient's acceptance of the visual outcome and the use of his or her previous correction. Has he or she been wearing spectacles only, if at all? Has he or she ever been fully corrected for the refractive error, or has the correction been reduced? If he or she has worn contact lenses, were the lenses rigid, soft spheres utilizing a *spherical equivalent* (or *masking*), or torics (and if so, what design)?

If a patient has not worn toric lenses previously, the visual correction may be surprisingly and dramatically different. For example, an individual who presents with acuities of 20/40, yet is correctable to 20/20, is usually dramatically surprised by (but unable to tolerate) the drastic improvement in vision. Be conservative in toric correction; most patients can tolerate an astigmatic undercorrection with complete satisfaction.

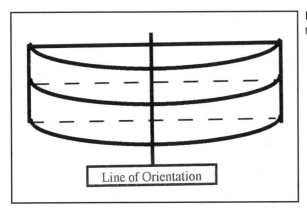

Figure 6-1. Line of orientation or axis of the cylinder.

Line of Orientation

In determining which toric alternative would best suit the patient, a flow chart approach is recommended. The patient's needs and other factors are listed, along with the type of lens(es) that fit those criteria (Tables 6-1 and 6-2). Then, a reference source is needed for finding out what is available. There are several such references available such as *Tyler's Quarterly, Contact Lenses and Solutions Summary,* and *Review of Optometry: Annual Contact Review.* In addition, manufacturers' fitting guideline booklets and customer service lines can be utilized.

Evaluating the Astigmatism

The major refractive question is whether the astigmatism is corneal and/or lenticular. This is ascertained by subtracting the CA as measured with the keratometer, from the manifest astigmatism (MA) as measured via refractometry. The resulting difference is referred to as internal residual astigmatism (IRA). The formula is IRA = MA – CA.

To define the difference between corneal and lenticular astigmatism (IRA), the refractometrist needs to utilize a combination of objective and subjective measures. Objective measures include retinoscopy, keratometry, or corneal topography. The subjective measure is the refraction and determination of best visual acuity and quality. The IRA is then simply the difference between the objective and subjective, remembering to take into account vertex correction for the subjective refraction.

Masking

Next, what is the patient's sensitivity to full cylindrical correction? Cylinder sensitivity should be determined prior to fitting (see Chapter 3).

The spherical equivalent (masking effect) is often applied to low cylinders of -0.75 or less. (Unfortunately, some clinicians attempt this method on moderate to high cylinders. This is not recommended.) Masking is accomplished by using a significantly thicker hydrogel or a low water content lenses due to their rigidity (or lack of deformity). This will have a small minus tear layer effect, correcting approximately 0.50 diopters of corneal cylinder.

This author traditionally corrects low cylinders with an astigmatic lens when the patient demonstrates sensitivity to the cylindrical correction. If masking or spherical equivalence is utilized, the clinician should perform a spherocylindrical over-refraction to determine if the patient appreciates the difference in visual quality.

Uncorrected cylinder in soft contact lenses depends on the design used to fit the patient. Often a low cylinder of 0.25 DC to 0.50 DC may be reduced and not appreciated in an over-refraction

Table 6-1.
Lens Design Options

Flourosilicone Acrylate	Hybrid Design*	Hydrogel
a. Moderate to high Dk	a. Limited to low Dk	a. High water, toric
b. Back or bitoric design	b. Satisfies corneal cylinder only	b. Back or front toric
c. Distance vision only	c. Distance vision only	c. Distance vision only
d. Monovision	d. Monovision	d. Monovision
e. Bifocal	e. Over-correction for uncorrected astigmatism	

Hybrid implies a soft/gas permeable lens, such as Softperm. Hybrid lens designs are limited to correcting corneal cylinder only.

Table 6-2.
Corneal/Refractive Astigmatism and Lens Selection

Amount of Refractive Corneal Cylinder	Lens Choice
Low (< 0.67 DC)	Spherical equivalent or masking lens (masking: high rigidity or prism base-down)
Moderate (0.75 to 2.50 DC)	Front or back toric prism ballast or double thin zone (consider frequent replacement)
High (x > 2.75 DC)	Front or back toric, custom, or rigid bitoric
Low (< 0.67 DC)	Spherical equivalent
Moderate (0.75 to 2.50 DC)	Front or back toric with ancillary spectacles, rigid bitoric more appropriate
High (x > 2.75 DC)	Front or back toric with ancillary spectacles, rigid bitoric more appropriate

when using thicker and/or low water content lenses. However, when ultra-thin and/or high water content lenses are used, the refractive astigmatism *will* be appreciated in over-refraction. Astigmatic hydrophilic lenses are available in low cylinder, starting at -0.75 DC. These lenses should be considered when fitting astigmatic patients. Generally, with-the-rule refractive errors are less sensitive to uncorrected cylinder than are against-the-rule and oblique, respectively.

OptT

Hydrogel Astigmatic Lens Design, Selection, and Fitting Methods

An astigmatic diagnostic fit should not be more complicated than a standard hydrogel fit. The lens design should be based on the type of astigmatism. A keratometric reading equal to the refractive cylinder and no greater than 0.67 DC could be fit with a spherical equivalent or masking lens. In cases of moderate cylinder (0.75 to 2.25), a hydrogel of either front or back design is satisfactory. If the astigmatism is significantly higher (> 2.50 DC), a custom toric design would need to fabricated. However, in higher cylinders, a hybrid or bitoric rigid is probably more appropriate.

Deciding which lens will serve as a good choice for the first diagnostic trial can be simplified by using a criteria table. The criteria table should be developed to address the refractive and ker-

Table 6-3.

Case History: Hydrogel Toric, 42-Year-Old Patient, -6.00 – 3.00 x 040

Lens Name	BC: 8.6 or 8.7	-5.50 DS	-2.25 DC	40° + 8° (32°- 48°)	Flexible Wear	Planned Replacement	Order of Choice
Optifit 3 (Wesley Jessen)	X	X	X	X	X		3°
Spectrum (Ciba)	X	X		X	X		4°
Optima FW (B & L)	X	X		X	X	X	3°
Sunsoft Toric or Eclipse	X	X	X	X	X		2°
Hydrocurve 3 Toric: PBH	X	X			X		5°
Focus Planned Replacement	X	X		X	X	X	2°
Preference Planned Replacement	X	X	X	X	X	X	1°
Gold Medallist Planned Replacement	X	X	X		X	X	3°
Specialty Ultavision T-FRP	X	X	X	X		X	2°
SunSoft Planned Replacement Multiples	X	X	X	X	X	X	1°
FreshLook Disposable Toric	X				X	X	6°
Soflens 66 Toric	X			X	X	X	6°
Coopervision Hydrasoft Options	X	X	X	X	X	X	1°

Criteria required for this case:
A. Keratometry: 42 (8.03)/44 (7.67) at 130, -2.00 x 040, clear and regular mires
B. IRA = MA – CA = -1.00 DC
C. Cylinder sensitivity: tolerates +0.75 DC, ±8° axis rotation.
D. Based on vertex correction: the contact lens (hydrogel *Rx*) should be approximately -5.50 – 2.50 x 040
E. Lens parameters required: 8.6/8.7 BC, - 5.50 – 2.25 x (32° to 48°)
F. Flexible wear versus conventional or planned replacement

atometric requirements as well as the patient's desired lens wear and replacement schedule. (See example, Table 6-3.) Diagnostic lens evaluations should be performed. An appropriate and inexpensive diagnostic set of lenses would be ±2 or 3 diopter spheres with -1.50 diopter cylinder at axes 45, 90, 135, and 180. Another option is to obtain "plano -2.00" and "plano -3.00" lenses (at the same axes) and perform a spherocylinder over-refraction. This over-refraction should be biased to the spherical component more so than the cylindrical component. These small diagnostic sets allow the clinician to observe the lens on the eye and determine, prior to ordering, the appropriate power and axis for the soft toric lens. If a diagnostic set of lenses are not available, many manufacturers have generous trial lens policies which allow for a diagnostic trial lens to be ordered at a negligible cost.

Ordering a lens without performing a diagnostic fit is referred to as an *empirical fit*. Empirical implies that the lens is ordered based on the known examination findings as well as assumptions on how the lens may perform on the eye in regards to lens rotation and axis stability.

Greater than 82% of all astigmatic hydrogel lenses can be fit empirically, meeting clinical and subjective tolerances of axis orientation, subjective visual acuity, and quality. Therefore, one may assume a safety zone in certain empirical fits; yet it is best to trial fit a diagnostic lens closest to axis and to power prior to ordering.[1,2]

A diagnostic fit will allow an assessment of a patient's tolerance for a lens, as well as an evaluation of the lens fitting relationships. A diagnostic lens allows the clinician to determine the axis orientation, coverage, movement, and comfort with a particular lens design in order to make the appropriate compensations.

Axis Adjustments

Prior to ordering the lens, a Cylinder Sensitivity Test[3] should be performed in order to determine the patient's sensitivity to lens torsion and/or under-corrected cylinder. This is easily accomplished in a trial frame and is highly recommended prior to the selection of a diagnostic lens. The test utilizes the principle of a "Just Noticeable Difference" (JND) or "first appreciable blur."

The cylinder sensitivity test is as follows.

1) Place the full manifest refraction in a trial frame. (This is preferred over the use of a phoropter.)

2) Isolate the best line of acuity that the patient has achieved. (Note: Moderate to high astigmatism may not achieve 20/20 and may have a form of amblyopia in that meridian.)

3) Slowly rotate the cylinder axis until the patient notes a change (JND) in visual quality. Note the amount of rotation.

4) Return the lens system back to the original axis, and repeat step 3 in the opposite direction.

5) Return the lens system back to the orginal manifest axis and reduce the cylinder in 0.25 diopter steps until there is a noted JND in visual quality.

6) Reduce the trial frame cylinder to the JND measurement and repeat the axis rotation test.

All hydrogel toric lenses have markings to indicate the position of axis and ballasting (prism weight at the bottom of the lens). These may be two lines at 3 and 9 o'clock on the front lens surface, a single droplet or line at 6 o'clock, or a series of three lines at the inferior margin of the lens (either as a color imprint or angled apart by 15 or 30 degrees) (Figure 6-2). These orientation marks assist the examiner in predicting the possible misalignment of the toric axis. When examining the lens with the slit lamp, imagine that the lens is the face of a clock. Each five-minute block on the clock is equivalent to a 30 degree lens rotation.

The LARS (left add/right subtract) principle implies that if the lens rotates *left*, the compensation would be to *add* the estimated number of degrees to the subjective axis. If the lens turns *right*, then one should *subtract* the number of degrees from the subjective axis. The LARS principle applies to both hydrogel and rigid front toric designs (Figure 6-3).

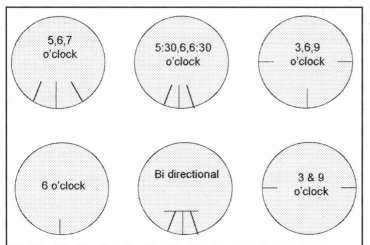

Figure 6-2. Toric orientation marks.

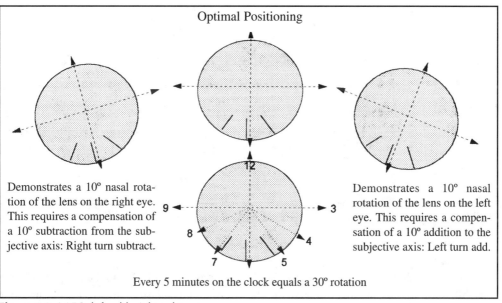

Optimal Positioning

Demonstrates a 10° nasal rotation of the lens on the right eye. This requires a compensation of a 10° subtraction from the subjective axis: Right turn subtract.

Demonstrates a 10° nasal rotation of the lens on the left eye. This requires a compensation of a 10° addition to the subjective axis: Left turn add.

Every 5 minutes on the clock equals a 30° rotation

Figure 6-3. LARS: left add, right subtract.

Lens Stabilization

Rotational stability, otherwise known as dynamic stabilization, is maintained in the toric lens design by either prism ballast, truncation, thin zones, or peri-ballast (Figure 6-4).

Prism ballasting utilizes approximately 0.75 base-down to 1.50 base-down prism with a base apex line at 90° to 270° (vertical). Prism ballast adds additional lens mass to the inferior portion of the lens while thinning the superior portion of the lens. Base-down prism relocates the center of gravity inferiorly thereby forcing the lens to have less rotation against gravitational and lid influences.

Truncation of a toric lens is a form of prism ballast enhancement. It has a profile analogous to that of a flat tire. A truncated design is a lens with an inferior portion of approximately 1.0 mm to 1.5 mm of material removed. Truncation forces the lens to settle inferiorly on the lower cornea. The lens then interacts with the lower lid such that the lid acts like a stop or brake.

OptA

OptA

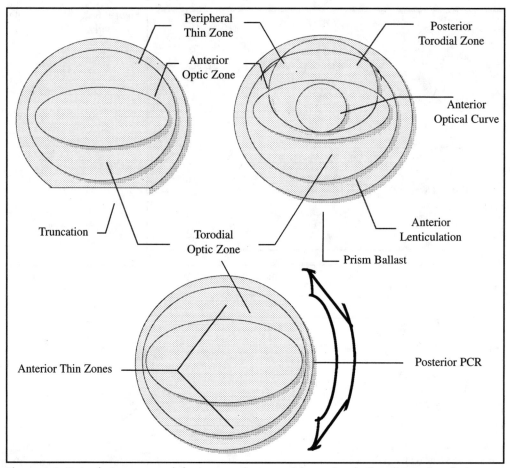

Figure 6-4. Toric designs, upper left—truncated, upper right—prism ballast (lenticulated), lower—thin zone (double slab-off).

OptA

Truncation allows the lens to position parallel to the inferior lid. Due to the peripheral thickness difference of plus and minus lenses, the amount of prism ballasting involved with truncation will vary. The prism ballast required for a minus lens is greater than that needed for a plus lens. A minus lens will also be lighter when material is removed, versus a plus lens, requiring additional prism to offset the weight loss.

Thin zones, referred to as the "Watermelon Seed Effect," are another form of rotational stabilization. A thin zone design reduces the peripheral thicknesses of the inferior and superior porions of the lens. This in turn reduces lid interaction, allowing the lens to be wedged between the upper and lower lids. With the incorporation of the thin zones, the center gravity is maintained at the geometric center.

Peri-ballast is a design that has an increasing lens thickness without peripheral edge tapering or thinning. The lens design is generally lenticulated with superior thinning and a thicker, weightier inferior ballast. This is not physiologically advantageous, however. Additional peripheral thickening can induce changes related to hypoxia, such as neovascularization. (This problem can occur with standard prism ballast.)

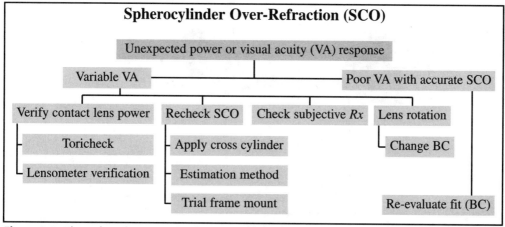

Figure 6-5. Flow chart for poor visual acuity with hydrogel torics. (Adapted from Myers RI, et al. Using over-refraction in soft toric fitting. *International Contact Lens Clinic.* 1990;17(9/10):233.

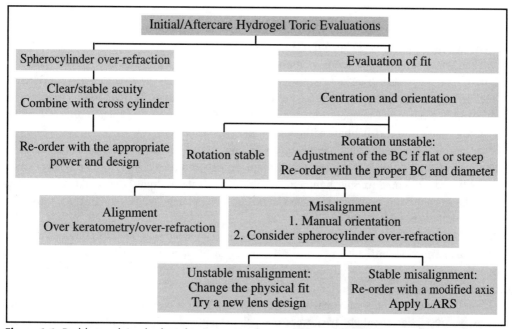

Figure 6-6. Problem-solving hydrogel toric contact lenses. (Adapted from Eiden SB. Precision management of high astigmats with toric hydrogel contact lenses. *Contact Lens Spectrum.* June 1992;43-49.

Problem-Solving Soft Toric Contact Lenses

The most common problems associated with soft toric lenses are related to vision and comfort (Figures 6-5 and 6-6). Comfort complaints are primarily due to an increased lens awareness related to increased lens mass and thickness, while lens displacement and/or torsion causes a reduction in visual acuity.

Lens dehydration is a major culprit for reduced comfort and acuity. When a lens dehydrates it will start to vault away from the corneal surface and will tend to lock out of its proper posi-

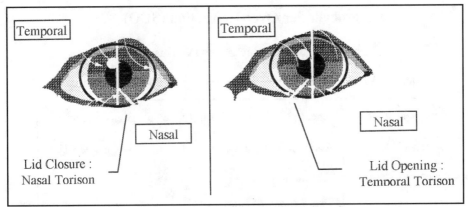

Figure 6-7. Nasal and temporal torsion effects induced by lid closure.

tion. The proper use of wetting drops will prevent lens dehydration and subsequent lens steepening, allowing the lens to maintain a proper lens/cornea alignment, thus enhancing comfort and visual stability.

Alternately, variable acuity may occur because the lid is forcing the lens to rotate (nasally on lid closure and temporally on opening) (Figure 6-7).

The patient should be asked if vision is stable or variable throughout the day. If vision is blurred, is it constant or transient? Transient blurring implies that the lens may have a flat BC, which is easily remedied by using a steeper BC. However, a steeper BC may have a tendency to stay fixed in the nasal or temporal orientation or to vault away from the apical cornea. In either of these situations, the visual blur will become more persistent.

A constant blur implies that there is either an uncorrected refractive error or a constant misalignment of the lens axis. If the lens is misaligned, it should be placed into its proper position manually and monitored for misalignment after blinking. If it misaligns after blinking, the lens is flat and a steeper BC is required. If it stays in position, the patient needs to be instructed to manually align the lens after insertion.

The lens should also be monitored for clinical signs of steepness, such as conjunctival congestion and infection, difficult lens removal, and/or induced apical distortions due to vaulting. If the lens appears to have induced rotation without proper re-orientation, the BC may need to be flattened to allow for increased freedom of movement.[5]

Another cause of constant blur with a hydrogel toric lens is residual cylinder. A spherocylindrical over-refraction should be performed on each patient with the lens in its proper orientation. Such an over-refraction will likely produce an oblique crossed cylinder. There are several methods to determine the final power for the contact lens when there is a significant spherocylindrical over-refraction. The trial frame method is simple and quick. Simply place the known contact lens power into a trial frame. Then place the trial lens equal to the spherocylinder over-refraction in the same trial frame. Place the trial frame on the lensometer and read the resultant power. (This method takes into account misalignment of the soft toric lens.)

Rigid Gas Permeable Astigmatic Contact Lenses

There are numerous methods for correcting astigmatism with rigid gas permeable lenses. The main problem in rigid lens fitting is the presumed difficulty in lens design. However, rigid lens-

Table 6-4. Base Curve Selection Based on Corneal Cylinder		
	Corneal Cylinder	BC Selection (for minus lenses)
Low cylinder	Plano to -0.50 DC	0.50 to 0.75 D flatter
	0.75 to 1.00 DC	0.25 to 0.50 D flatter
Moderate cylinder	1.25 to 1.50 DC	On K to 0.25 D flatter
	1.75 to 2.00 DC	0.25 D steeper
	2.25 to 2.50 DC	0.50 D steeper
High cylinder	2.75 to 3.00 DC	0.50 to 0.75 D steeper

For plus lenses, fit the BC 0.25 to 0.50 steeper than recommended for minus lenses

Adapted from Morgan BW. RGP material selection and design. EyeQuest. 1994;2:49-58.

es allow the clinician to become a "contact lens tailor." Keep it simple. Design the lens with respect to the corneal topography and refractive error (Table 6-4).

Low to Moderate Toric Corneas: Spherical Designs

When the corneal toricity is low (-0.25 to -0.75 DC) a spherical lens design can be used. The goal of this design is to create an alignment with the corneal surface. As the corneal toricity increases, the lack of alignment decreases. This would suggest that a toric design is required.

When designing a spherical lens for a low toric cornea, the BC should match the flat keratometric reading. This will create an alignment with the flat meridian and allow for a tear lens effect throughout the steep meridian (Figure 6-8). The tear lens will act as a cylindrical lens, correcting the majority of the corneal cylinder.

Once the lens is inserted, specific fluorescein patterns will be observed based on the form of CA (see Chapter 5, Fluorescein Patterns).

Moderate to High Astigmatism

When corneal toricity becomes significantly greater than 2.00 DC, various toric lens design alternatives should be considered such as back surface torics (saddle fit, low toric simulation) or bitoric design. The goal of a toric lens design is to match the back surface of the lens to corneal topography and each meridian of power.

Back Toric Lenses

The same basic principles of rigid lens design apply to back surface toric designs. Back surface lens designs are preferred when corneal cylinder is moderate to high and there is an absence of lenticular or residual astigmatism. BC measures are generally selected "on K" or "flatter than K" (Figure 6-9). While this design rarely provides adequate visual acuity due to the tear/lens effect, it is very useful when the induced cylinder equals the amount of uncorrected subjective cylinder.

A back toric is used when the induced cylinder will equal the amount of uncorrected subjective cylinder. (For example, suppose the patient had a refraction of -0.50 – 3.00 x 90 with keratometry of 43 @ 90/44.50 @ 180 (yielding -1.50 diopters corneal cylinder at axis 90). In this case, the residual cylinder is half of the total refractive cylinder.) Back toric lenses are used to get rid of cylindrical powers based on an "induced cylinder" effect of material and on index of refrac-

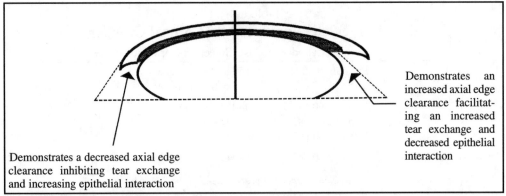

Demonstrates a decreased axial edge clearance inhibiting tear exchange and increasing epithelial interaction

Demonstrates an increased axial edge clearance facilitating an increased tear exchange and decreased epithelial interaction

Figure 6-8. Axial edge clearance: tear exchange and epithelial interaction.

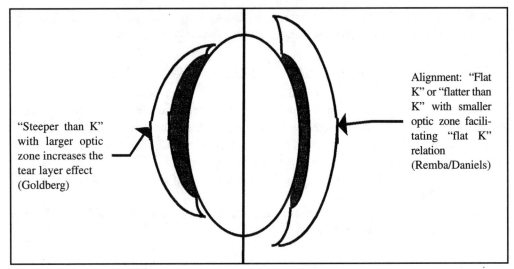

"Steeper than K" with larger optic zone increases the tear layer effect (Goldberg)

Alignment: "Flat K" or "flatter than K" with smaller optic zone facilitating "flat K" relation (Remba/Daniels)

Figure 6-9. Tear layer/optic zone relation in back torics.

tion differences. This requires several calculations that can be simplified by multiplying the subjective cylinder by -0.456. If the result is close to the amount of residual cylinder power, a back toric is the lens of choice. The lens is then ordered with a spherical vertex-corrected power in a back toric design.

Saddle Fit

A saddle fit establishes a full alignment to the two principle meridians. A "fit on K" design for each meridian will get rid of any corneal cylinder, but will create a tight lens fit. The saddle fit requires a smaller optic zone. It will tend to fit intra-palpebrally with a slight lid attachment. A saddle fit will yield adequate cylindrical correction if there is an absence of lenticular astigmatism.

Low Toric Simulation

The low toric simulation design is based on an intended undercorrection of the corneal cylinder. The design essentially converts a high cylindrical power to a moderate cylinder. The result is a fit that is looser than the saddle fit, but similar to a spherical equivalent.

Low toric simulation design mimics a flatter (and thus looser) fit. The design uses a "flatter than K" fit for the flat meridian and undercorrects the steep meridian by approximately one-third. For example, a low toric simulation lens being used for a 44/47 cornea would be fit as 43.50/45.50. This would be equivalent to 0.33 x 3 DC, which would equal a 2 DC back surface correction. The additional compensation for the uncorrected cylinder can be made by increasing the OZD. This allows for a slight increase in the tear film effect.

Bitoric Rigid Lens Design

The bitoric lens design is highly favorable in many cases of moderate to high amounts of CA particularly if there is lenticular astigmatism. The bitoric lens is essentially a back surface toric designed to be flatter in each meridian with an additional compensating front toric correction. The bitoric lens design is advantageous in that it fits the two major corneal meridians (due to its back surface toric design). That is, the cylinder on the front surface corrects residual astigmatism and the cylinder on the back surface corrects CA. It possesses an optical quality similar to a spherical lens, and has no induced tear lens effect. Furthermore, acuity will not be affected by lens rotation.

Fitting bitorics can be made simple by using a set of diagnostic lenses. The set varies in BC selection and usually comes in a 2 or 3 DC series. Using such a set allows for a straightforward spherocylinder over-refraction and better certainty that the first lens order will be optimal.

If a bitoric diagnostic lens set is not available, the fitter may either use spherical lenses for a basic diagnostic fit or design the lenses empirically. The use of a spherical lens can be accomplished in one of two ways:

Method 1. Assess a spherical rigid lens of a BC equal to the flat keratometric value plus 20% of the corneal toricity. For example: "flat K"= 44 (7.67), "steep K"= 47 (7.18), so corneal toricity = -3.00. The diagnostic lens selection would equal: 20% (or 0.02) x -3.00 = 0.60 diopters or 44.60 (7.56). Then perform a spherocylinder over-refraction.

Method 2. Assess a "flat K" lens on each meridian. The BC of the lens to be ordered should be flattened to achieve an alignment pattern in each meridian.

Mandell and Moore[6] have developed a simple guideline in designing bitoric lenses. The premise to a bitoric design is to simply think of each meridian separately. A spherical lens will be designed for each meridian with a fit factor that will flatten the BC in order to avoid the tear lens effect. Generally, the flat meridian is fit 0.25 diopters flatter than k while the steeper meridian is fit 0.50 to 1.25 diopters flatter, based upon the amount of corneal cylinder. The flattening in the steeper meridian will be 0.50 to 1.25 diopters progressing from 2.00 corneal cylinder and up, respectively.

For example, -6.00–3.00 x 040, keratometry equal to 42 (8.03) / 44 (7.67) x 040 clear and regular mires, and MA–CA = IRA (plano -1.00 dc x 040). A back toric lens design would leave the patient under-corrected for IRA, therefore a bitoric lens design should be designed using the methods described in Tables 6-5 and 6-6, and Figure 6-10.

Table 6-5.
Fit Factor

CORNEAL CYL.	STEEP MERIDIAN	FLAT MERIDIAN
2.00	0.50 flatter	on K
2.50	0.50 flatter	0.25 flatter
3.00	0.75 flatter	0.25 flatter
3.50	0.75 flatter	0.25 flatter
4.00	1.00 flatter	0.25 flatter
5.00	1.25 flatter	0.25 flatter

Adapted from Mandell RB, Moore CF. A bitoric lens guide that really is simple. Contact Lens Spectrum. *November 1988;4(11).*

Table 6-6.
Bitoric Lens Guide

Keratometry	42 (8.03) @ 130			44 (7.67) @ 040
Spectacle refraction		-6.00 -3.00 x 040		

		Flattest K	Sphere Power	Steepest K	Sphere + Cyl. Power
1	Enter K	42 (8.03)		44 (7.67)	
2	Enter spectacle power		-6.00		-9.00
3	Vertex correction		-5.50		-8.00
4	Fit factor	(-).25	(+).25	(-).75	(+).75
Add lines	Add lines	1 & 4	3 & 4	1 & 4	3 & 4
5	Final CL Rx	41.75 (8.08)	-5.25	43.25 (7.80)	-7.25

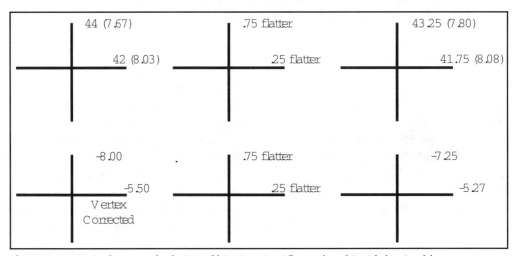

Figure 6-10. Optical cross calculation of bitoric using "flatter than k" with lacrimal lens compensation, and the basic rule 0.05 mm = 0.25 D

References

1. Myers R, Jones D. Can soft toric lenses be empirically fit? *Optical Prism.* January 1992:34-37.

2. Ames KS, Erickson P, Medici L. Factors influencing hydrogel toric lens rotation. *International Contact Lens Clinic.* 1989;16(7,8):16-21.

3. Becherer PD. Management of astigmatism with soft toric contact lenses. *Practical Optometry.*1993; 4(4):168-170

4. Tomlinson A. Succeeding with toric soft lenses. *Review of Optometry.* July 1983;7:72-80

5. Rakow PL. Problem solving with toric hydrogels. *Contact Lens Forum.* November 1990:29-36.

6. Mandell RB, Moore CF. A bitoric lens guide that really is simple. *Contact Lens Spectrum.* November 1988;4(11):83-85.

Patient Instructions for Handling Lenses

- Proper patient education is crucial to a successful contact lens fit.

- Teach the patient to become comfortable touching the eye prior to insertion and removal (I & R) instruction.

- Teach the patient to always wash the hands before handling lenses.

- To decrease lens loss, teach the patient to cover the work area with a towel.

- Before insertion, the lenses should be inspected for debris, tears, chips, etc.

- Teach the patient to check his or her vision after lens insertion.

Introduction

Proper education and reinforcement of correct lens insertion and removal (I & R) as well as lens care are critical to a successful fit. Each aftercare visit should re-address the patient's techniques of both I & R and lens care. Complacency and poor compliance are the two major culprits in complications related to contact lenses. If the patient is well educated on the proper techniques, it is less likely that he or she will have serious problems. A videotape or pamphlet is quite helpful in explaining the proper procedures. A checklist of procedures should be reviewed with the patient prior to and after training. The checklist can also act as a "report card," identifying areas that require further training or attention.

What the Patient Needs to Know

- Cosmetics should be applied *after* lens insertion.

- Cover your eyes when using any type of hair spray.

- Washing the hands is the most important aspect of lens handling and lens care.

- Do not use lotions, creams, deodorant soaps, or oils that may coat the lens.

- Never expose your contact lenses to saliva or tap water.

- Use the specified care products only.

- Avoid touching the contact lens with the fingernails.

- Before placing the lens on the eye, inspect it for defects and tears.

- Re-hydration of a dried-out soft lens will not sufficiently restore the lens. The lens should be discarded.

- If the lens becomes dislodged or dislocated, examine the eye in a mirror to locate the lens. If the lens cannot be located (and if the lens was not dropped or lost) report to your doctor.

- If the lens is difficult to remove or if there is an increased sensitivity upon lens removal, your lens may be too tight. This should be reported to your doctor.

- If the eye becomes red, swollen, or uncomfortable, if your vision is blurred, or there is a discharge, remove the lens immediately and report to your doctor right away.

A contact lens agreement form should be used as a contract between the doctor and the patient. This form should identify that the fitter has reviewed I & R techniques and has advised the patient of any possible adverse reactions.

Preparing for Lens Insertion

Have the patient prepare the working area by placing a white towel on the counter top. (Working over a sink or in free space often leads to lens loss.) If the lens is dropped in a sink or on the floor, it should be cleansed prior to re-insertion. The patient may want to invest in a small magnification mirror to make lens I & R easier.

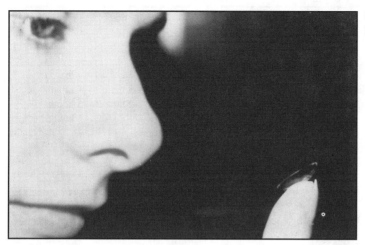

Figure 7-1. Soft contact lens inspection.

Lens handling starts with proper hygiene habits. Set a good example and wash your hands in front of the patient prior to the handling of any contact lens product. Instruct the patient to *always* wash the hands prior to lens handling. When drying the hands, a lint-free cloth or towel is advisable. Avoid soaps with oils and lanolins or the use of cosmetics or creams/lotions prior to lens handling. Cosmetics should always be applied *after* lens insertion.

To ease any apprehension, the patient should be taught to touch the eye prior to any lens training. Instruct the patient to wash the hands and then rest the thumb on the cheek and middle finger on the lower eyelid. The patient is instructed to gaze upward and place the index finger onto the lower bulbar conjunctiva. This mimics lens insertion. To become familiar with lens removal, have the patient press the index finger and thumb together mimicking a set of tweezers. Have them reach up and grasp the medial portion of their lower eyelid.

Prior to lens insertion, instruct the patient to remove the lens from its storage case. The patient should take note that the lens is properly immersed in its storage solution. The lens can be rinsed with saline or a multi-purpose soft lens solution, but should never be immersed or rinsed in tap water. (Tap water carries a high volume of bacteria that can be easily transferred to the eye.) The lens should then be inspected for any defects, tears, chips, debris, or deposits (Figure 7-1).

Wear Schedules

The patient's eye will need to adapt to lens wear. An abbreviated lens wear schedule should be prepared for the patient based on the type of lens he or she will be wearing. There are two lens adaptation schedules that are recommended (Table 7-1).

Handling Soft Lenses

Many soft lenses are thin and difficult to handle. The patient should be instructed to grasp the lens between the thumb and index finger and draw it along the side of the index finger. This will remove excess fluid so that the lens can be properly inspected. This is also helpful when trying to determine lens inversion (that is, whether or not the lens is inside out).

Lens inversion is determined in three ways. The first method is to place the lens on the top of the index finger and view it by looking across the lens surface. If the lens is inverted, the top edge

Table 7-1. Adaptive Lens Wearing Schedules			
Schedule One		**Schedule Two**	
Day 1	4 to 5 hrs on	Day 1	3 hrs on—3 hrs off—4 hrs on
Day 2	5 to 6 hrs on	Day 2	4 hrs on—3 hrs off—4 hrs on
Day 3	6 to 7 hrs on	Day 3	5 hrs on—2 hrs off—5 hrs on
Day 4	7 to 8 hrs on	Day 4	5 hrs on—1 hrs off—5 hrs on
Day 5	8 to 10 hrs on	Day 5	10 hrs on
Day 6	8 to 10 hrs on	Day 6	10 hrs on
Day 7	8 to 10 hrs on	Day 7	10 hrs on

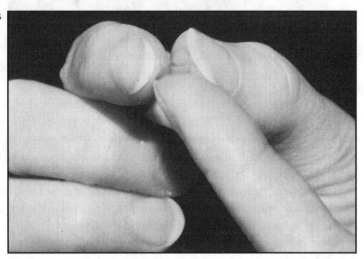

Figure 7-2. Taco test for lens inversion.

of the lens will appear to be bowed flat and flared out. If the lens is turned the right way, the lens edges will appear upright pointing upward like a bowl.

The second method is called the "Taco Test" (Figure 7-2). Grasp the slightly dry lens from the edge and observe how it curls. The lens will be bowed outward (like a potato chip) if inverted. If the lens is turned the right way the lens will appear to roll inward onto itself similar to the shape of a taco or cannoli (whatever your stomach desires!).

The final method is incorporated during manufacturing. Some companies have placed an inversion marker or indicator on the lens surface, usually the initials of the company name. The indicator should appear as a "WJ" or "AV" (depending on the brand of lens) on the outside of the lens if is in its proper position. The marker will appear as "JW" or "VA" if the lens is inverted.

Lens Insertion Technique

It is recommended that the new lens wearer use two hands to insert the lens. The patient is instructed to hold the upper lid taut in order to keep the lashes away from the lens as follows:

1) Place the lens on the index finger of the dominant hand (Figure 7-3). (Generally, the right lens is inserted first.) *Note:* It helps to dry the finger first. A wet lens will be attracted to a wet cornea. If the finger is wet, the lens will stay on the finger.

2) Using the same hand, place the thumb on the cheek for support and place the middle finger onto the medial lid margin.

3) Place the other hand above the head with the fingers pointed down to the medial upper lid.

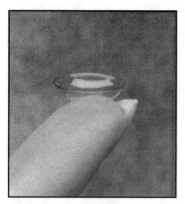

Figure 7-3. Soft contact lens position for insertion.

Place the middle finger on the medial superior lid margin and pull upward towards the bony rim of the eye.

4) The lower and upper lids are pulled apart simultaneously to expose a large ocular working space. Place the lens onto the bottom portion of the eye or directly onto the cornea with gentle pressure (Figure 7-4a and b).

5) Touch the lens onto the eye with gentle pressure and roll the finger temporally to allow the lens to release from the finger.

6) While holding the upper and lower lid, slowly look down into the lens while lightly pushing the lens up with the lower lid.

7) Prior to releasing the lid, look at the lens in a mirror to assure that the lens is properly placed. Also look for any air pockets.

8) To help center the lens, close the lids and lightly massage the upper lid.

9) Repeat with the second lens.

The lens may be slightly uncomfortable immediately upon lens insertion. This can occur due to acidic care products, residual peroxide, foreign matter underneath the lens, improper insertion technique, dehydrated lens, or lens defects. The majority of these problems can be easily solved by irrigating with wetting drops (without removing the lens from the eye). Another option is to leave the lens on the eye, but slide the lens over onto the sclera and "swirl" it around with the finger. If this doesn't solve the problem, remove the lens and irrigate.

Removal Technique

Lens removal is the most important technique the patient must learn. If the lens is uncomfortable or the eye becomes red, the lens needs to be removed. It is advisable to place a wetting drop on the eye to re-hydrate the lens and allow it to become buoyant prior to removal. To remove the lens:

1) Place the middle finger onto the lower lid margin in order to control lid action.

2) Place the other hand above the head with the index finger pointed down to the middle of the upper lid. Place the middle finger on the middle of the upper lid edge and pull upward towards the bony rim of the eye.

3) The lower and upper lids are pulled apart simultaneously, exposing a large ocular working space.

Figure 7-4a. Soft contact lens insertion.

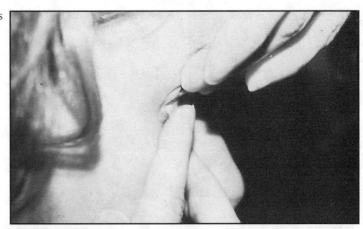

Figure 7-4b. Soft contact lens insertion by fitter.

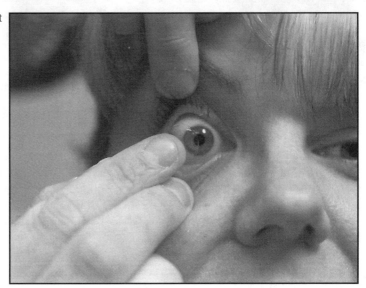

4) The index finger is placed onto the bottom of the contact lens. With gentle pressure, pull the lens down towards the bottom of the eye.

5) Reach inward with the thumb. The lens is pinched between the index finger and thumb at the 6 o'clock position (Figure 7-5a and b). This will break any surface attraction between the contact lens and the cornea, allowing for easy removal.

Lens Care

When cleaning soft lenses, it is advisable for the patient to work with the lens in the palm rather than between the fingertips (Figure 7-6a and b). The patient should place an ample volume of cleaning solution into a *cupped* palm and work the lens in a circular fashion (Figure 7-7). (Cleaning in a flat palm allows the lens to dehydrate, which will increase its fragility. Maintaining the lens in a wet state will decrease the incidence of lens damage.) Cleaning systems will be covered in the next chapter.

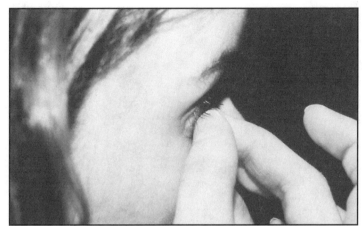

Figure 7-5a. Soft contact lens removal.

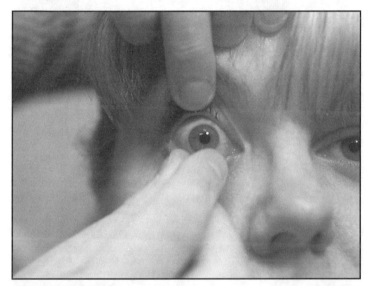

Figure 7-5b. Soft contact lens removal by fitter.

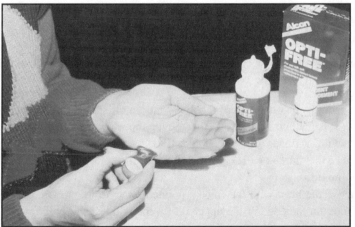

Figure 7-6a. Soft contact lens cleaning.

Figure 7-6b. Soft contact lens cleaning in open palm.

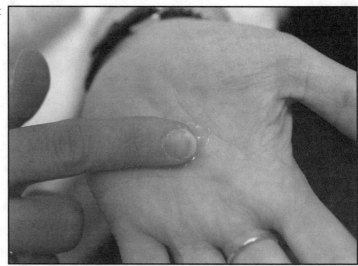

Figure 7-7. Soft contact lens cleaning in closed palm. This is the preferred method.

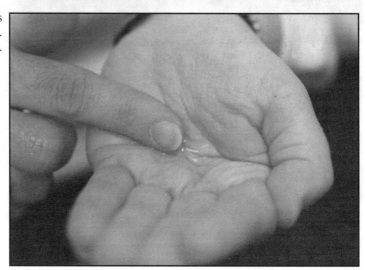

Handling Gas Permeable/Rigid Lenses

To remove the lens from the case, fill the container with an ample supply of storage solution so that the lens floats. Slide the lens up the wall of the case and onto the fingertip, then inspect it for defects and/or adherent debris.

Lens placement technique requires that the upper lid be held taut in order to keep the upper lid lashes away from the lens. (This method is similar to that taught above for soft lenses.)

1) Place the right lens on the index finger of the dominant hand.

2) Using the same hand, place the thumb on the cheek for support, then place the middle finger onto the middle of the bottom lid.

3) Place the other hand above the head with the fingers pointed down to the middle of the upper lid. Place the middle finger on the edge of the upper lid (in the middle) and pull upward towards the bony rim of the eye.

4) The lower and upper lids are pulled apart simultaneously to expose a large ocular working space. Place the lens directly onto the cornea with gentle pressure (Figure 7-8).

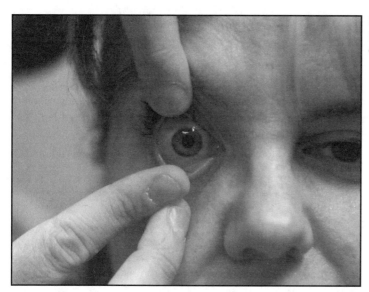

Figure 7-8. Placement of rigid gas permeable lens on eye by fitter.

What the Patient Needs to Know

- Do not use aerosol products when wearing contact lenses. If you are in the area of an aerosol product, shield your eyes or wear safety eyewear.

- Avoid wearing lenses where there are fumes, irritating vapors, dust, or smoke.

- If you work in a laboratory, check Occupational Safety and Health Association (OSHA) regulations to determine if contact lenses are forbidden.

- Do not wear lenses in swimming pools, hot tubs, steam rooms, or during water sport activities.

- If you are hospitalized, contact lens use should be discontinued.

- Lenses should be discontinued if you are undergoing immunosuppression treatment.

- Do not use eye drops (except approved re-wetting drops) with the contact lens on the eye. Eye medications should be administered *prior to* insertion *or after* the removal of contact lenses.

- Apply makeup *after* inserting your lenses.

- Remove your lenses *before* removing makeup.

- If daily wear lenses are prescribed, do not sleep with the lenses inserted overnight. (Short naps may be safe if you use wetting drops when you wake up…ask your doctor.)

- If you are wearing rigid lenses, always close your eyes if you must wipe them.

- Maintain a regular aftercare schedule with your eye doctor at the suggested intervals.

5) Prior to releasing the lid, look at the lens in a mirror to assure that the lens is properly placed on the eye.

6) Repeat with the left lens.

If the patient has difficulty with lens insertion due to hand tremors or fixation problems, a suction cup can be used to assist in lens placement. The lens is moistened with conditioning solution and gently placed onto the holder (without exerting suction). Then the lens is placed onto the cornea as if the lens were on the index finger. While the average patient should not be encouraged to use the device on a regular basis, certain patients (such as aphakes) will have to depend on this method.

Lens Recentration

Occasionally, rigid lenses will become decentered onto the bulbar conjunctiva or underneath the lid. This most often happens with new patients who are not properly performing lens insertion or who are blinking prior to full lens placement onto the cornea. When the lens dislocates onto the conjunctiva, it will tend to bind due to the lack of curvature conformity. This can be quite alarming to the patient. Therefore, recentration of the lens must be taught during the initial training.

To recenter the lens, the patient must first locate the lens on the eye. This can be done by looking into a mirror or feeling the lens through the lids. The lens should then be slid to the temporal or bottom part of the eye. Next, the lens is held in place with gentle pressure on the most temporal or inferior position. This slightly lifts the opposite side of the lens from the eye's surface. The lens can then slide up and over the corneal surface as the patient moves the eye toward the lens.

Lens Removal

Two hands are generally required to remove a rigid lens. The technique is as follows:

1) Use the index and middle finger to grasp the upper and lower lid. (The lids need to be sufficiently separated in order to expose the entire cornea.)

2) The lids are pulled back and tightly against the eye so that the lids come behind the edges of the lens (Figure 7-9).

3) Blink. This will force the lid margins to come into contact with the lens edge, expelling the lens. The opposite hand should be cupped under the eye in order to catch the lens.

The most important part of this technique is to open the lids wide enough while still keeping them taut against the eye.

Another method of lens removal is to use a suction cup. This is not a preferred method except for those individuals who have dexterity problems. First, the suction cup is moistened with a drop of lubricating fluid. The patient is to keep the head upright while using a mirror to locate the lens on the eye. The cup is then guided towards the lens and brought squarely onto the lens with light pressure. As the lens makes contact with the cup, the stem of the holder is released, which will create a suction between the lens and the cup. The lens can then be easily lifted off of the eye.

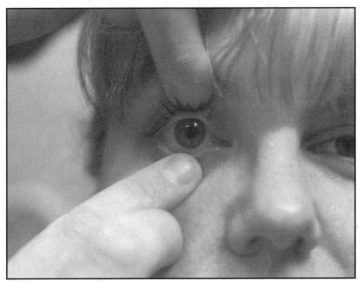

Figure 7-9. Rigid gas permeable lens removal by fitter.

Parting Comments

Precautions can be summarized by saying, "After lens insertion, you should have consistently sharp vision, the lenses should remain comfortable, and your eyes should stay white." The vision should be checked upon lens insertion. Instruct the patient to check the vision of each eye individually; it should remain at the same level each day. The lens should achieve an optimal level of comfort within a few minutes after lens insertion.

Finally, the patient should be told to look into a mirror periodically to inspect the appearance of the eyes. If the eyes appear red while wearing the lens(es), wetting drops should be instilled. If wetting drops do not relieve the redness, the lens should be removed. If the eye clears after removal, there is a good chance that the lens was defective. If the eye stays red after lens removal, the patient should be instructed to report to the doctor.

Chapter 8

Care Product Systems

KEY POINTS

- The components of a care product system remove excess debris, remove protein film, and kill potentially destructive bacteria.

- Rinsing agents are used to remove lens debris and loosely adhered bacteria.

- Daily cleaners cleanse the lens surface and reduce the majority of bacteria.

- Disinfection completes the bacteriocidal effectiveness of the system, particularly against resistant bacteria.

- Additional surface cleansing can be accomplished via enzymatic action that will hydrolyze adherent tear proteins.

- Contact lens cases may be a source of bacterial contamination and should be replaced monthly.

Introduction

Components of a care product system are designed to reduce the majority of bacteria, reduce bacterial colonization, and reduce the protein film on the lens. This is accomplished by incorporating daily cleaners, rinsing agents, disinfectants, and enzyme products.

What the Patient Needs to Know

- Always wash your hands before handling the lenses.

- Do not skip your prescribed daily cleaning and disinfecting routine.

- Do not skip a step in the cleaning and/or disinfecting process.

- Maintain a clean lens case.

- If you drop your lens onto a countertop, floor, or sink, you MUST clean and disinfect it again before placing it on your eye.

- Do not touch the bottle tips to the lenses, your hands, or any other surface.

- Do not put bottle caps rim-down on counter tops or other work surfaces.

- Do not mix and match products. Stick with the brand that your doctor has suggested.

- If your eyes sting and/or get red when you put your lenses in, remove the lenses at once. If the problem resolves once you've removed the lens, you may rinse the lens with saline and re-insert. However, if the problem recurs, remove the lens and notify your eye doctor.

Elements of the Care System

Daily Cleaners

The effectiveness of a system depends on adequate daily cleaning. This is generally done by applying the cleaner to the lens as the lens is held in the cupped palm. The lens is then gently rubbed with a finger.

Daily cleaners are either surfactants, abrasives, or solvents, any of which enhance the effectiveness of digital cleaning (Table 8-1 and Figure 8-1).

Rinsing Agents

Rinsing agents remove excessive debris and bacterial colonies from the lens after cleaning. In order to maintain stability, buffering agents and chelators are added to these products. The buffering agents may have additional cleansing effects, but may discolor certain lenses. Chelating agents are used to remove loosely adhered debris, to reduce the potential toxicity of residual chemicals from care products, and to enhance the detergent cleansing ability of the product. Preservatives are sometimes added in order to prolong product shelf life. However, the incorporation of preservatives may demonstrate a higher incidence of hypersensitivity reactions. Rinsing products have a pH (acid-base) range of 7.0 to 7.4, versus the normal tears' pH of 7.2.

Table 8-1.
Types of Daily Cleansing Agents

Type of Cleaner	Method of Cleaner	Action of Cleaner	Precautions
Abrasive	Polymeric bead to rasp across the lens surface	Enhances mechanical cleaning and disrupts surface film	Shake before using
Solvent	Isopropyl alcohol or peroxide	Denatures proteinacous film and dissolves lipids and fats	Does not require added preservatives. May cause surface defects with rigid gas permeable materials
Surfactant	Non-ionic mechanical emulsifier or detergent	Uses a micelle (or soap) to disrupt surface film. Contains surface active agent that attaches itself to surface debris	

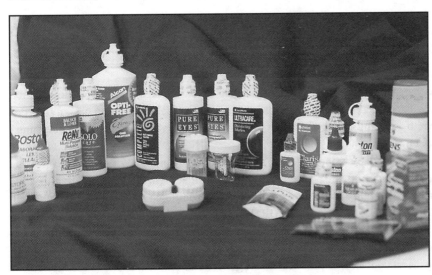

Figure 8-1. A complement of care products for both rigid gas permeable and soft contact lenses.

Saline, a popular rinsing agent, is available as preserved or non-preserved in large multiple-use bottles and single-dose units, as well as in aerosol containers. Aerosol containers can be preservative-free, but may demonstrate an acidic shift over time. Secondly, aerosols require a propellant to expel the solution that, at times, may not be efficient.

Disinfection

After the completion of daily cleaning and rinsing, the lenses must be disinfected. Disinfection is the process where vegetative or living microorganisms are killed, although spores may survive. Spores are capable of germination (growth), allowing for future contamination. A disinfectant protects against infection by killing microbes, viruses, and fungi. (In contrast, sterilization means *killing* microbes, including their spores.)

At present, thermal or heat systems only disinfect, they do not sterilize. Heat disinfection depends on proper manual cleaning and rinsing, otherwise it is possible to "bake" on debris and inadequately reduce bacteria colonization. Heat can also reduce the lens' water content, negatively affecting the parameters of high water content lenses. Combination chemical and heat systems have fallen to a minimal market share and will not be further discussed in this chapter.

Enzymatic Cleaners

Additional surface cleansing can be accomplished via enzyme action that hydrolyzes adherent tear proteins. Enzyme cleaners contain either papain, pancreatin, or subtilisin. Each of these products must be dissolved in saline or peroxide. Several manufacturers have introduced a liquid enzyme for daily enzymatic cleaning to be used with preservative-based systems, such as OptiFree or OptiOne (Alcon Laboratories, Fort Worth, Tex), or they have incorporated an enzymatic component, such as with Renu Plus (Bausch & Lomb, Claremont, Calif). These systems are highly recommended for disposable and frequent replacement hydrogel lenses.

Weekly enzyme cleaning is extremely valuable for durable or conventional lenses. In contrast, enzyme use can be minimized with disposable lenses. This is because the frequency of replacement means that there is usually a lack of significant protein build-up on the lens surface. Heavy depositors should utilize weekly or daily enzyme cleaners and/or increase their rate of lens replacement.

Chemical Care Systems

The various care product systems presently available on the market incorporate a rinsing agent, a daily cleaner, and a disinfectant product. The ultimate goal of a system design is to promote compliance by making the care product system safe and easy to use while maintaining a high level of effectiveness (Table 8-2).

Thimerosal is a mercury compound used as a topical antiseptic and/or preservative. It is a slow-acting agent that lacks broad-spectrum activity, but is highly effective against gram-positive bacteria. To enhance its ability, it is often combined with additional preservatives or enhancers such as ethylene diamine tetra-acetic acid (EDTA). Approximately 5% to 8% of patients are hypersensitive to thimerosal. Patients exhibiting hypersensitivity will present with ocular injection, conjunctival chemosis, photophobia, foreign body sensation, and/or diffuse superficial punctate keratopathy. Most contact lens products no longer contain thimerosal due to the high rate of allergic reactions.

Chlorohexidine digluconate is a germicide preservative used only in rigid lens products; it is not used in soft lens care products due to its ability to bind to the hydrogel matrix. It also has the potential to interact negatively with epithelial cells. Chlorohexidine is not effective against encapsulated microbes. This agent can also cause hypersensitivity reactions, presenting primarily as dermatitis or similar manifestations as seen when using thimerosal.

Benzalkonium chloride (BAK) is a quaternary ammonium that is effective against both gram-positive and gram-negative microbes. BAK has a weak affinity for binding to PMMA and rigid gas permeable materials; however it has a high affinity for hydrogel polymers. BAK (in sufficiently high levels) is toxic to corneal tissue. Allergic reaction can occur, but due to its wide use in many hygiene and cosmetic products, most individuals have been desensitized.

Sorbates, or sorbic acid, have an antibacterial and anti-fungal effect and are incorporated as enhancing agents in contact lens saline. Sorbates will often cause a yellowing of hydrogel polymers. Sorbic acid does not cause hypersensitivity reactions; however, some patients may complain of a "stinging" sensation due to an acidic shift in the solution.

Table 8-2.
Adverse Reactions and Lens Changes Associated with Care Products

Complications	Cause/Etiology
Corneal staining	1. Improper combination of products 2. Thimerosal products used concurrently with tetracycline 3. Insufficient rinsing of daily cleaner 4. Insufficient removal of enzymatic cleaner 5. Insufficient neutralization of peroxide 6. Storage in benzalkonium chloride
Acute red eye	1. Preservative hypersensitivity 2. Insufficient neutralization of peroxide 3. Inadvertent mixing of sorbate or chlorohexidine with quaternary ammoniums
Ocular irritation	1. Insufficient rinsing of daily cleaner 2. Insufficient neutralization of peroxide 3. Hypersensitivity to preservative agents 4. Acidic or alkaline shift in care product pH 5. Use of non-buffered agents 6. Debris on lens surface on insertion 7. Insufficient removal or rinsing of enzymatic residue
Lens parameter changes	1. Excessive peroxide exposure 2. Heating lenses in chemical disinfectants

Lens discoloration	1. Gray/Black: thimerosal used with thermal units
	2. Yellowish/Brown:
	  a) use of sorbate-containing products
	  b) excessive proteinacous coating
	3. Yellow/Green: use of standard sodium fluorescein
	4. Opaque:
	  a) use of chlorohexidine with thermal disinfection
	  b) use of expired care products
	  c) switching from chemical to thermal disinfection without purging
	  d) heating with products of a high viscosity

Fading of tinted lenses	1. Use of solvent-based products 2. Use of benzoyl peroxide (ie, acne preparations)
Incompatibilities	1. Generic hydrogen peroxide 2. Mismatching of products can lead to instability and ineffective disinfection. 3. High water content parameter changes using thermal disinfection 4. Polyquad is not compatible with sorbic buffers
Lens dryness	1. Improper digital cleaning 2. Improper use of enzymatic cleaner 3. Improper use of oil- and/or lanolin-based hand cleaners and lotions
Rigid gas permeable surface defects	1. Exposure to alcohol cleansers 2. Excessive polishing at high speeds 3. Excessive digital pressure, inducing lens warping

Adapted from Wesibarth RE, Ghormley NR. Hydrogel lens care regimens and patient education. In: Bennett E, Weissman BA, eds. Clinical Contact Lens Practice. *Philadelphia, Pa: JB Lippincott; 1991.*

Table 8-3. **Peroxide-Based Disinfecting Systems**			
Method of Neutralization	**Reduction**	**Chemical Reaction**	**Residual Peroxide**
Platinum disk neutralization	Reduces peroxide to isotonic saline and oxygen	Catalytic reaction peroxide with platinum yields isotonic saline	5 to 15 ppm
Time released neutralization	3% peroxide for 18 to 20 minutes, leaving a residual peroxide concentration	A hydroxypropyl methyl-cellulose (HPMC) coating encapsulates the catalase tablet. Enzymes reduce peroxide to isotonic saline.	5 ppm
Dilution system	Serial dilution of peroxide with saline	Dilution requires several steps to reduce the concentration of the peroxide.	200 ppm

Polyaminopropyl biguanide and polyquaternium are quaternary ammoniums. The large diameters of these molecules prevent them from being absorbed into the lens polymer. They are non-toxic, non-irritating, non-sensitizing, and effective against both gram-positive and gram-negative microbes. They are slow-acting, weak preservatives. There is a low incidence of adverse reactions. These preservatives are used in single-step care products to clean, rinse, and disinfect.

Hydrogen peroxide-based systems rely on exposing the microorganism to a harsh oxidative condition. Peroxide creates a disruption between the internal and external environment of the microbial cellular walls and membranes. Exposure time requires a minimum of 10 minutes followed by a neutralization time of 20 minutes to 4 hours (Table 8-3). Hydrogen peroxide has the ability to destroy all major pathogens related to contact lens wear. It has a rapid antimicrobial activity and is able to eradicate fungi within 1 hour. Additionally, peroxide is highly effective against *Acanthamoeba* cysts within 48 to 68 minutes. It is also very effective against HIV.

Hydrogen peroxide disinfection requires a neutralization of the peroxide into saline. The basic concept behind all peroxide-based systems is for disinfection and neutralization to proceed concurrently. This adds to patient convenience and better compliance, while avoiding the use of potentially toxic preservatives.

Isopropyl alcohol has a significant bacteriocidal and solvent cleansing ability, making it ideal for a simplified care product. A combination of isopropyl alcohol and a surfactant cleaner demonstrates antimicrobial activity acceptable to FDA standards. Alcohol-based systems are effective against 95% of *Acanthamoeba* cysts, as well as HIV. However, alcohol-based products are too harsh for rigid gas permeable lenses, causing brittleness and subsequent cracking.[1]

Future of Lens Care Systems

Chlorine is presently utilized in Europe, but has not been approved in the United States. Chlorine demonstrates an optimal antimicrobial activity. However, it exhibits significant ocular incompatibility, as evidenced by conjunctival injection.

Ultrasound cleans lenses by surface disruption using a process called cavitation. Cavitation causes bubbles to suddenly form and collapse on the lens surface. To maximize the bacteriocidal effect of ultrasound, lenses can be submerged in a compatible disinfecting solution. This system would allow a "hands-free" cleaning and disinfection; it would be easy to use, and presumably increase compliance.

References

1. Roseman MJ, Hill RM. Aerobic responses to the cornea to isopropyl alcohol measured in vivo. *Acta Ophthalmol.* 1987;65(10):306-312.

Lens Verification and Modification Techniques

- Quality assurance demands that you verify the parameters of a lens before dispensing.

- Parameters to be verified include power, BC, diameter, curve diameters, and CT.

- Baseline measurements of lens parameters should be made *prior* to proceeding with any modification.

- Minimize the amount of modification in order to prevent lens damage.

- If a lens requires multiple modifications, it should be sent back to the lab.

Lens Verification

Fitting lenses is one thing; knowing what you are fitting is another. Even though the lab requires a quality assurance inspection of the contact lens prior to shipment, the office should also assure that the order meets specifications.

Power Verification

Contact lens power can be verified on a lensometer in the same way as spectacles (Figure 9-1). The lensometer should be placed into a vertical position so that the lens sits freely on the lens stop. (If the lens is held between the fingers, subtle pressure can cause optical distortion and a misrepresentation of the lens power.) A rigid lens should be clean and dry, then placed convex side up to measure the back vertex lens power (Figure 9-2). (The lens stop should have a reduced diameter of approximately 4 mm so as not to lose or drop the lens.) The front vertex lens power is measured by placing the lens concave side up (Figure 9-3). Front vertex power is usually measured only on high plus lenses.

When verifying the power of a toric rigid lens, the mire image will appear sharp and distinct at two different powers. If the lens is warped, an indistinct second mire will appear. A toric lens will have power measurements exactly 90 degrees apart, while the power readings of a warped lens will be greater or lesser than 90 degrees apart. Front toric lenses should be measured in a minus cylinder format, but will need to be decentered due to the prism incorporated into the lens design.

Hydrogel lens power can also be verified by lensometry. The lens is placed on a fiber-free cotton towel and blotted dry, then placed on the lens stop using forceps. The lens should be centered and measured three times to verify power. (Hydration of the lens plays a major role in the validity of the measure.) If a toric lens is to be measured, place the lens on the lens stop with the inferior lens mark at 6 o'clock. The two power measures should be 90 degrees apart.

A second method of hydrogel lens power verification is the use of a wet cell, a small chamber that can be filled with saline. The cell is placed onto the lens stop. When using a wet cell, one must multiply the measured power by 4.6 in order to compensate for the indices of refraction of the lens and saline. (For example, if the measured power equals -1.00, the actual power would equal -4.60.)

Base Curve Measurements

The determination of the BC is as important as the measurement of power. The BC can be measured by several methods, the most common of which is the radiuscope.

The lens mount for the radiuscope has a concave countersink in which the lens is placed. The BC is measured as follows (Figure 9-4):

1) A drop of saline is placed into the well of the lens mount (Figure 9-5). The dry lens is placed onto the mount convex side down (Figure 9-6).

2) The stage and lens mount of the radiuscope are then aligned so that the light source (usually green) projects into the center of the lens.

3) The eyepiece is focused with the power adjusted to zero. At this point the inspector will see a "spoke-like" image.

4) The stage of the scope is adjusted so that the spoke-like image aligns with two peripheral/diagonal lines inside the scope. Once these are aligned, the gross power knob is turned toward

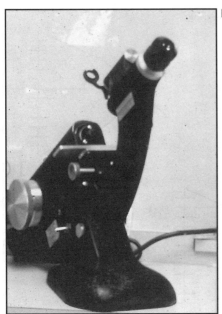

Figure 9-1. Power inspection: lensometer (vertexometer).

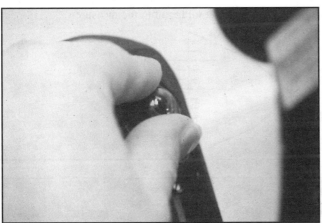

Figure 9-2. Measuring back vertex power.

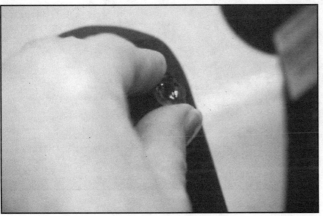

Figure 9-3. Measuring front vertex power.

Figure 9-4. Measuring with a radius-cope.

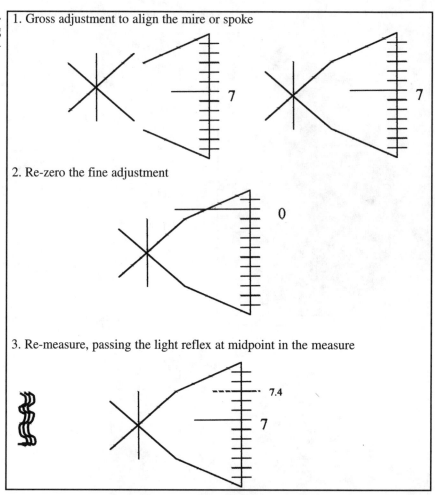

1. Gross adjustment to align the mire or spoke

2. Re-zero the fine adjustment

3. Re-measure, passing the light reflex at midpoint in the measure

Figure 9-5. Placement of saline on lens mount.

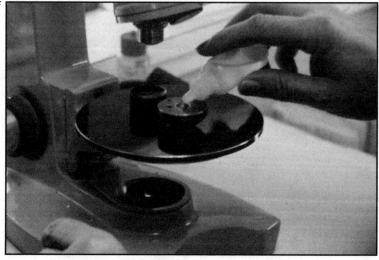

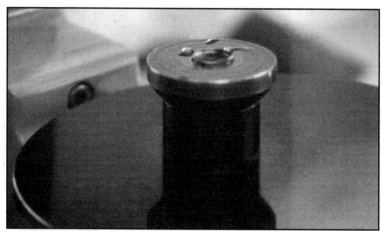

Figure 9-6. Lens placement on a lens mount.

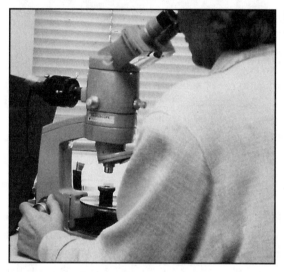

Figure 9-7. Gross adjustment of radiuscope: approximate BC and reticule alignment.

the higher ranges (Figure 9-7). The viewer will notice a serrated image of the light source (resembling a coil) at the midpoint of the curvature range.

5) Continue turning the gross adjustment until the second spoke-like image is seen.

6) Re-adjust the spoke image so that the diagonal lines of the image meet evenly with the diagonal lines of the measure scale on the right side.

7) Turn the gross focus back to zero. Adjust the fine focus line measure to zero (Figure 9-8).

8) Turn the gross focus as you did in steps 4 through 6.

9) The final curvature is read from the scale (on the right side of the viewer) to the nearest hundredth of a millimeter.

A toric BC must be differentiated from a warped lens. A warped lens will not exhibit a distinct second image. It will appear as a spoke-like image in which some of the spokes are consistently out of focus as compared to the remaining spokes, but are not 90° apart. A toric lens will demonstrate an image with one meridian in focus and the opposite meridian, 90° away, distinct-

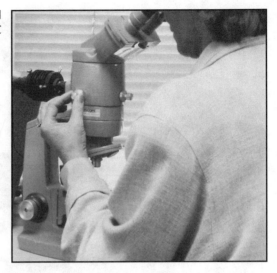

Figure 9-8. Fine adjustment: establishes final reticule alignment and zeroing prior to final BC measurement.

ly out of focus or blurred. If unsure, lensometry can be used to differentiate a warped from a toric lens. (This will identify whether or not the meridians are 90° apart.)

The most convenient method for BC verification is a template matching system. This system works for both rigid and hydrogel lenses, but is more efficient for hydrogels. The lens is placed onto a mount that has convex surfaces of predetermined curves. If the lens is steeper than the template, a bubble will appear in the center portion of the lens. If the lens is flatter than the template, the lens will not center or will standoff from the template.

OptA Linear Dimensions

The overall lens diameter, OZD, and PCR widths can be measured by several devices. A pupillary distance (PD) stick, 7x loupe, V channel, or a projection magnifier are all acceptable measuring devices limited only by the magnification available. The magnification loupe and the projection magnifier can be used with both hydrogel and rigid lenses. The only variability is that the hydrogel lens needs to be measured in a wet state. This is accomplished by using a wet cell mount on the projection magnifier.

The overall lens diameter can be measured several ways. The simplest method (and least accurate) is the PD stick. The lens can be placed directly onto the PD stick and measured from edge to edge. A second method (for rigid lenses) is the V Gauge or V channel, a device similar to a ruler with a v-shaped channel down the middle (Figure 9-9). The lens is dropped down into the channel and measured at the point it becomes lodged.

The most accurate method of measuring lens diameter is to use a 7x or 10x magnifying loupe (Figure 9-10). A reticule is etched into the faceplate on which the lens is placed, so that the edge of the lens is at zero (Figure 9-11). The overall diameter is measured by simply looking across the linear rule. Individual PCRs can also be measured on this device. Simply move the lens so that the inner curves, which appear slightly blurred, are aligned with the zero mark on the reticule. The lens can be inspected for surface quality at the same time.

An equivalent type of device is the projection magnifier, a desktop device that has a greater level of magnification for a proper inspection and lens measure.

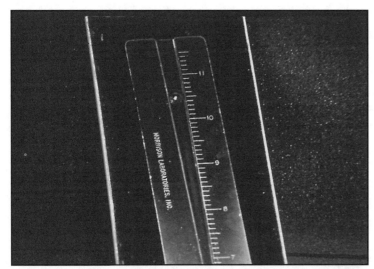

Figure 9-9. V gauge for measuring lens diameter.

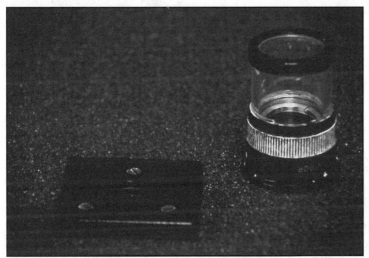

Figure 9-10. 7x loupe and lens mount.

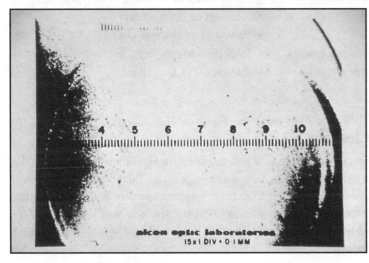

Figure 9-11. Reticule of loupe.

Center Thickness (CT)

The CT for rigid gas permeable lenses is easily measured by using a thickness gauge (Figure 9-12). This gauge has a small mount for the lens. Once the lens is placed on the mount, a plunger-type rod is gently lowered onto the lens (Figure 9-13). The measurement is based on the separation created by the lens between the mount and the tip of the rod. The rod is attached to a clock gauge that is numbered in millimeter increments.

For soft lenses, an ultrasonic pachymeter can be used to measure the thickness of the lens. Take a measurement of the corneal thickness alone. Then place the contact lens on the eye, and gently repeat the measurement. The difference between the two measurements will equal the soft lens thickness.

OptT

Lens Modification

Modification procedures are easy to learn but require practice. There are limitations to modifications associated with the lens material. PMMA materials can easily withstand multiple modification techniques. However, rigid gas permeable lenses with silicone and/or fluorine can easily be distorted by numerous modification procedures. The fitter should minimize the amount of modification in order to prevent lens damage. If a lens requires multiple modifications, it should be sent back to the lab. Baseline measurements of lens parameters should be made *prior* to proceeding with any modification.

The modification unit is a simple system with a small electrical motor mounted in a portable or desktop box (Figure 9-14). The motor has a spindle that protrudes up into a plastic or stainless steel catch bucket or splash tube. The motor spins between 700 to 1200 revolutions per minute (rpm). A lower spin rate is required for silicone and fluorinated lens materials. (To prevent excessive heat buildup or lens warping, rates of 300 to 500 rpms are preferred for fluorinated materials.)

Modification tools are mounted onto the spindle via a male-female system. Tools to polish, edge, and refinish curves include:

- Cut-down tool or stone
- 90 degree cut-down tool or stone
- Polishing tools (8.4, 9.00, or 10 mm)
- Polishing compound
- Diameter gauge
- Double-sided tape (cloth attachment)
- Lens holder with spinner
- Sponge tool
- Bevel tool or stone
- 90 degree polishing or cone tool
- Three-inch flat polishing disk
- Suction cup (lens holder)
- Velveteen or chamois cloth
- Inspection loupe (7x)
- Radii tools (7.6 to 12 mm)

Lens Polishes and Cleaners

There are several commercially available lens polishes used for rigid lens modification. The polishes are composed of tin oxide or calcium carbonate compounds. The purpose of the polish is to prevent heat buildup that could warp or burn the lens. Ample amounts of polish with a splatter of water or the use of contact lens wetting solution of higher viscosity will keep the surface of the tools moist during modification procedures. The tool is covered by a soft fabric or padded material to which polish is applied.

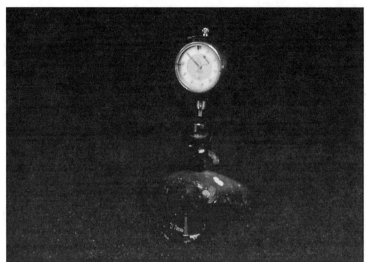

Figure 9-12. Thickness gauge.

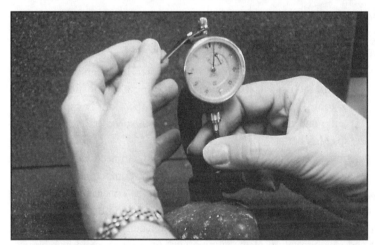

Figure 9-13. Placement of lens and measurement of lens thickness.

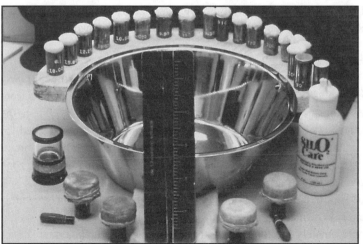

Figure 9-14. Rigid gas permeable modification unit.

If the patient describes vision problems with a lens, inspect the surface for dry spots or residual manufacturing pitch. Cleaning the lens will rectify many of these problems. However, some surface debris cannot be easily removed with standard cleaners. More resistant deposits need to be removed with solvent-type cleansers, which are not available to the public. The solvent cleanser is used to degrade waxy build-up on the lens surface. A solvent cleanser may be an alcohol-based product such as Miraflow (Novartis-Ciba Vision, Atlanta, Ga) or QuickCare Starting Solution (Novartis-Ciba Vision, Atlanta, Ga). Another uncommonly used product is naphthane (lighter fluid). A quick cleaning with naphthane (less than 15 seconds) will more than adequately remove any waxy build-up. After using any form of solvent, rinse the lens thoroughly under tap water. After rinsing, apply conditioner to the lens in order to facilitate proper lens wetting. Polishing a lens with the unit is described later.

Peripheral Curve Fabrication and Blending

To incorporate and/or blend PCRs, one will need radius tools made of plastic or brass, or impregnated with diamond dust. The radii of these tools should range from 7.6 to 12 mm.

Peripheral Curve Modification

To perform curve modifications, select the proper radius tool and attach the velveteen cloth with waterproof double-sided tape or a high-tension rubber band. (The thickness of the tape and velveteen is about 0.2 and 0.4 mm, respectively. This must be accounted for when you select the radius tool. For example, if a 9.0 mm radius is desired, then an 8.8 mm radii tool should be used if using tape, or an 8.6 mm radii tool if using velveteen cloth.) After the cloth is applied, place the covered tool on the unit spindle and turn on the motor. Adjust the speed based on the lens material. Be conservative; less speed is better.

Mount the lens onto the suction cup (Figure 9-15). (The suction cup will need to be moistened with water to allow for proper lens suction.) Douse the cloth with polishing compound prior to introducing the lens to the tool. The lens should be held over the tool with the concave surface facing down. It is then gently placed onto the spinning tool. Rotate the suction cup in the opposite direction of the spindle spin. It is best to support the hand holding the suction cup with the opposite hand so that there is a consistent and steady rotation of the suction cup. In order to avoid lens burn or warpage, the lens should be lifted from the spindle every 5 to 10 seconds. If a spinner is used, hold the spinner at approximately a 45 to 60° angle away from the center point of the tool. It does not take long to fabricate a PCR, therefore the lens should be inspected after one or two applications.

Peripheral Curve Blending

A smooth or moderate blend will avoid adhesion, increase tear exchange, and allow for easy lens movement. The blending tool is selected based on the numerical average of the two adjacent curves. (For example, if the secondary curve is 8.0 mm and the intermediate curve is 9.0 mm, the proper blending tool is 8.5 mm.) As before, the curve of the blending tool must be adjusted for the thickness of the velveteen (and the tape too, if that is used vs. a rubber band). (One important note: never use a tool that is 0.5 mm or more flatter than the BC when blending the optic zone and the SCR. This may cause warping or an inadvertent increase in the OZD.)

Blending time should be kept to a minimum, otherwise the modification can change widths and diameter. Exposure time is equivalent to the amount of desired blend. Light blends should have an exposure time of approximately 5 seconds, medium or moderate blends should be 10 seconds, and heavy or smooth blends should be 15 to 20 seconds.

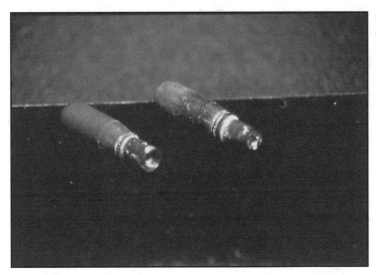

Figure 9-15. Suction cup/lens holder.

CN Bevels, Edge Contouring, and Polishing

One can shape, round, and taper the edge of the lens with several different techniques. The most common technique is the use of a 90 degree polishing or cone tool that can also be used to incorporate a CN bevel (Figure 9-16). (A CN bevel is an anterior tapering process to reduce thickness.) Edge modifications can also be completed using a sponge tool.

When performing a CN beveling or edge polishing procedure, the lens is mounted with the concave side of the lens on the suction cup (or the convex side facing the tool). The tool should be padded with velveteen, placed onto the spindle, and doused with polishing compound. The lens is introduced into the cavity of the tool perpendicular to the center of the tool. Do not force the lens into the tool, but allow the edges to lightly touch the inner cavity (Figure 9-17). The lens should be rotated opposite to the spindle rotation. Remove the lens from the tool and inspect it approximately every 10 seconds. This process will leave the anterior edge of the lens sharp, thus requiring the modifier to round and polish the edges.

Edge rounding and polishing can be easily performed with a conical or flat sponge tool (Figure 9-18). The lens is mounted concave side down on the suction cup or spinner device. Polishing compound is applied to the sponge. Touch the lens perpendicularly to the sponge tool for no longer than 10 seconds.

Surface Polishing

Surface polishing is used to cleanse the lens surface and remove deposits and scratches. The lens should first be inspected for surface integrity and the depth of scratches (Figure 9-19). If the scratches are severe, polishing will not improve the lens and the lens should be replaced. If the material has a high level of fluorination, minimize the polishing time to 5 to 10 seconds at a low rotation speed.

The easiest method is to use a hand polisher, which has a velveteen cloth or flat sponge mounted in a bracket that is held in the palm of the hand. Simply apply polishing compound to the pad. Using a figure-eight motion, move the convex surface of the lens across the pad with light to moderate pressure. Clean and inspect the lens (Figure 9-20).

Figure 9-16. 100 degree cone for front CN bevel (for peripheral edge lift).

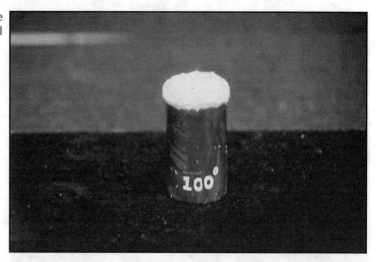

Figure 9-17. Placement of the lens into conical tool.

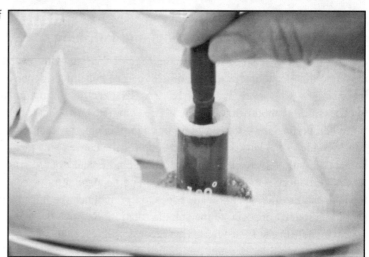

Figure 9-18. Lens edge rounding and polishing.

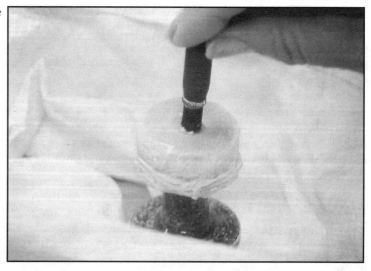

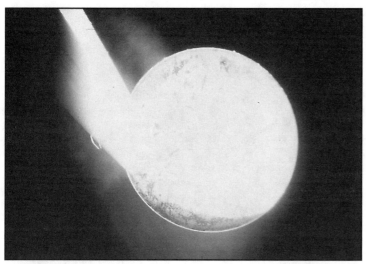

Figure 9-19. Lens prior to polishing.

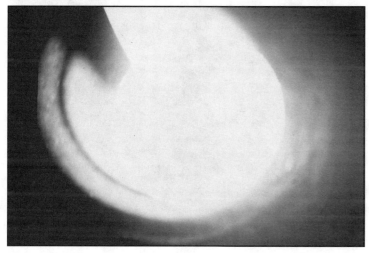

Figure 9-20. Lens after polishing.

A second method is to simply place polish on a cotton-tipped applicator. Or, place the lens on your fingertip and apply polishing compound to the lens surface. Gently rub the lens between the fingertips.

The third method uses the modification unit. The lens is placed onto the suction cup, convex side facing the tool (Figure 9-21). The flat sponge tool is placed on the unit spindle with an ample supply of polishing compound. The lens is placed gently onto the sponge at a 45 degree angle and rotated counterclockwise to the tool sponge. (The rotation can be accomplished manually or by mounting the lens on a spinner.) Hold the lens at an angle to polish the peripheral anterior surface. Polish the center portion of the lens by holding the lens perpendicular to the center of the sponge. Excessive pressure and polishing time could inadvertently create a power change in the lens, so be gentle and quick.

Concave surface polishing can be completed using the pad, cotton applicator, or fingertip method. If the modification unit is to be used, a conical sponge tool should be mounted on the spindle, and the lens should be mounted with the concave side facing the sponge (Figure 9-22).

Figure 9-21. Front surface polishing.

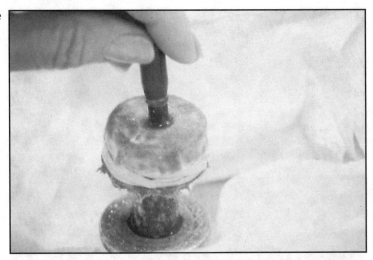

Figure 9-22. Back surface polishing.

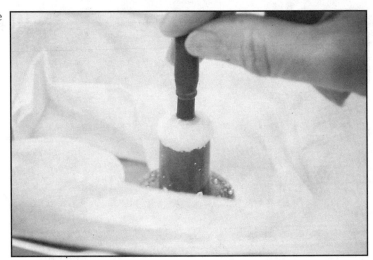

The lens is applied perpendicularly to the center point of the conical sponge with light pressure for approximately 10 to 15 seconds, based on the material.

Repowering a Rigid Lens

Repowering a rigid lens implies the addition or subtraction of fine increments of power to the lens by the removal of material from the center or the periphery (Figure 9-23). If one wants to add minus power to the lens, a small amount of central anterior lens flattening is required. If plus power is required, a small amount of peripheral material needs to be removed, thus increasing the front anterior curve. Caution should be taken in order not to distort or damage the lens. Repowering should be limited to adding ±0.37 diopters. *Excessive power changes to materials other than PMMA will only distort the lens optics.*

Adding minus is accomplished in the same manner as performing anterior surface polishing. The lens is mounted onto a suction cup with the convex surface facing the sponge tool or a con-

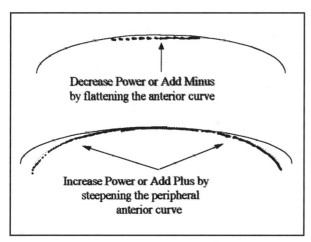

Figure 9-23. Lens repowering.

ical padded tool. Ample polishing compound is applied to the tool surface, then the lens is touched perpendicularly to the central portion of the sponge (or to the side of the conical padded tool). The application time should be brief and gentle. The lens should be removed from the suction cup and measured on the lensometer after each application.

The modifier must be more judicious in adding plus power. The flat sponge or conical padded tool can be used. In this scenario, the lens is held at an angle against the midpoint portion of the sponge tool or against the padded tool. The goal is to remove an adequate amount of anterior peripheral material in order to steepen the overall anterior curvature of the lens, thus increasing the plus power.

Chapter 10

Contact Lens Complications

KEY POINTS

- The majority of contact lens related complications of the cornea and conjunctiva are directly related to chronic hypoxia (lack of oxygen).

- The most common contact lens complications are due to difficult I & R, poor lens conditions (such as scratched lens surfaces or deposits), and the presence of debris on the back surface of the lens.

- Vascularization is the formation and extension of capillaries that had not previously existed.

- Subepithelial infiltrates (SEI) are secondary to an inflammatory reaction associated with chronic hypoxia, causing the aggregation of cellular components in the tissue.

- Corneal edema is due to the leakage of fluid into the cornea secondary to a change in the endothelial pump mechanism (which leads to a fluid influx into the stromal layer). Fluid leakage into the stroma results in central corneal clouding, striae, or folds.

- In giant papillary conjunctivitis (GPC) the surface of the palpebral conjunctiva, notably the upper lid, is covered with papillae. It is primarily an allergic reaction.

Introduction

Contact lenses are medical devices and should be treated with respect by the patient and the fitter. Complications associated with contact lenses can be anywhere from benign and annoying to severe and sight-threatening. Lack of patient compliance to proper wear schedules and care product use is often the major cause of contact lens-associated complications. However, the patient is not always at fault. Complications and adverse reactions occur for many other reasons, such as hypersensitivity to care products, reduced corneal oxygen delivery, bacterial colonization, or induced inflammatory response.

Physiological Aspects of Contact Lens Complications

Complications associated with contact lens wear are often directly related to chronic hypoxia (deprivation of oxygen) and subsequent corneal metabolic changes. This scenario induces cellular changes leading to the loss of cell strength, allowing an opportunity for bacterial infiltration and inflammation.

When there is a condition that causes oxygen deprivation or depleted conditions (ie, contact lens wear), a shift in the fluid balance of the cornea leads to edema. In its most basic terms, here's how that happens: 90% of the glucose (sugar) used by the corneal epithelium for energy is stored as glycogen. Under stressed conditions, corneal metabolism utilizes the stored glycogen to maintain cellular function. The by-products associated with the use of glycogen, such as lactic acid, cause a shift in the fluid balance of the cornea. The final effects of such acidosis lead to additional corneal structural changes, such as folds and striae.

Epithelial Complications Secondary to Contact Lenses

Micro-Mechanical Trauma

The most common contact lens complications occur as a result of difficult I & R and/or poor lens conditions (such as scratched lens surfaces, deposits, and the presence of back surface debris [BSD]). Dry lens surfaces will cause epithelial chafing, leading to a superficial trauma. This creates an opportunity for bacterial infiltration. This scenario is referred to as micro-mechanical trauma.[1]

Microcystic Edema

Definition: Microcysts are dead or aging cells trapped within the epithelium (Figure 10-1). They originate in the anterior basement membrane and are the direct result of increased carbon dioxide and acidosis. Microcystic eruptions occur at the superficial epithelial surface.

Observation: These eruptions are seen as discrete spots when stained with sodium fluorescein (staining may be minor to moderate), usually central to paracentral. They are best observed with retroillumination (30 to 40x). Under this lighting, the cysts appear in reversed illumination. Thus, the microcysts will appear dark on the same side of the light source and bright in the adjacent hemisphere of the microcyst. This is due to the higher index of refraction internal to the microcyst, associated with the accumulation of metabolic debris. The number of microcysts is documented as follows: 0 = None, 1 = 1 to 5, 2 = 6 to 25, 3 = 26 to 49, and 4 = >50.

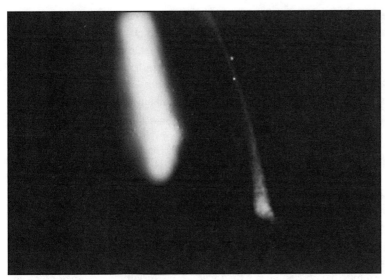

Figure 10-1. Microcysts.

Symptoms and Findings: The patient will generally be asymptomatic, although there may be a minor reduction in visual quality and acuity.

Treatment: If there are less than about 30 microcysts the condition requires no treatment, only monitoring. However, when there are greater than 30 microcysts it is recommended to decrease wear time and change to daily wear or high Dk rigid gas permeable lenses. The prognosis for the condition is good. After decreasing or ceasing wear, there will be a temporary increase of microcyst eruption with resolution in 5 weeks. If epithelial compromise is a concern, antibiotics are warranted.

Vacuoles

Definition: Vacuoles are gas- or fluid-filled intraepithelial pockets.

Observation: Vacuoles are small (20 to 50 microns) and round with distinct edges. They are best viewed with retroillumination, under which they will have an unreversed illumination. (Unreversed implys that the side of the vacuole closest to the light source is bright, while the opposite side appears dark.) This is because the gaseous content of the vacuole gives it a lower index of refraction, versus its surroundings. (This illumination is the exact opposite as seen in microcysts.)

Symptoms and Findings: Generally, patients are asymptomatic with minimal to minor reduction in visual quality and acuity, and minor to moderate punctate staining.

Treatment: This condition requires no treatment unless there is severe visual reduction (rare). If acuity is reduced, the patient should discontinue lens wear until edema resolves or visual acuity is stable. The prognosis is positive without long-term complications, allowing for the continuance of lens wear.

Back Surface Debris and Micro-Trauma

Definition: BSD is associated with metabolic waste, trapped cellular debris, and exogenous foreign bodies that get between the contact lens and the cornea, causing micro-mechanical trauma.

Observation: There is discrete punctate staining with moderate to severe depth. The appearance will be based on the depth of the impression made by the debris entrapped behind the lens.

Symptoms and Findings: The patient will have a variable range of discomfort with ocular injection. The symptoms will be proportional to the severity and depth of the induced defect. Discomfort will be mild to moderate (annoyance), with mild to moderate redness and visual acuity changes.

Treatment: The patient must temporarily discontinue lens use and be refit. The refit should address depositing characteristics and the effectiveness of care products. The lens should have proper centration, alignment without bearing, and lens movement to enhance tear fluid exchange. Prophylactic antibiotics may be required if there is a break in the epithelium. Patient education regarding lens hygiene is beneficial. The patient should use wetting drops on a regular basis, rinse the lens prior to insertion, and use the "scleral flush" technique to rid any entrapped debris. These steps will produce a dramatic increase in lens comfort and a decrease in ocular redness.

Vascular and Inflammatory Reactions

Definition: Vascularization is the formation or extension of capillaries that had not previously existed (Figure 10-2). Neovascularization is the formation of new vessels as an extension or shunt (connection) to pre-existing vascularization.

Etiology: Chronic hypoxia initiates the vascularization response. The lack of oxygen triggers lactate acidosis, which decreases the integrity of the epithelium and also causes stromal softening. This yields an opportunity for vessel ingrowth. In addition, inflammatory mediators are released during the early phase of vascularization. This stimulates additional vessel growth. Tight lenses, limbal compression, solution sensitivity, and/or trauma may also trigger the release of such inflammatory mediators with resulting vascularization.

Symptoms and Findings: Vascular responses to chronic hypoxia can vary from minor to severe based on whether or not there is also bacterial involvement. Corneal vascularization occurs in approximately 34% of cases associated with hydrogel lens use, versus 2% with non-lens wearers.

Observation: Vascularization looks like a mesh-like growth in the mid-epithelium, projecting towards the cornea like small spikes and/or branches called fronds. (These are different from normal limbal vessels which "loop" back towards the limbus.) Ninety eight percent of the vascularization occurs within the superficial stroma.[2] Low-grade (Grade 1) vessels tend to migrate inward approximately 0.6 mm (daily wear) to 1.4 mm (extended wear). Grade 2 migrates towards the pupil without passing into the pupillary zone; Grade 3 penetrates the pupillary region.

Additionally, intracorneal hemorrhage can occur due to the fragility of the new vessels. Such a hemorrhage will appear as a red spot on the cornea at the proximal end of a vascular frond. These hemorrhages should be monitored for spread. The patient should refrain from taking any medication that has an anticoagulant effect, such as aspirin.

Treatment: Treatment involves discontinuing contact lens use until the vessel(s) regress. After regression, ghost vessels (the abnormal blood vessels, now empty of blood) will persist. The patient can be refit to high water content hydrogel or high Dk rigid gas permeable lenses with sufficient axial edge clearance. Care products and lens schedules should be re-evaluated and patient education needs to be comprehensive. The patient should be monitored for re-vascularization.

Superior Limbic Keratitis/Vascularized Limbic Keratitis

Definition: Superior and vascularized limbic keratitis are limbal vascularized responses to chronic hypoxia associated with contact lenses. Superior limbic keratitis (SLK) is associated more with hydrogel lens wear (specifically, lens over-wear or chemical hypersensitivity such as thimerosal[3,4]) and vascularized limbic keratitis (VLK) more with rigid lens wear (specifically, larger diameters, low edge lift, and inhibited lens movement).

Observation:

SLK: There is an increase in the vascular response in the superior limbal/bulbar conjunctiva

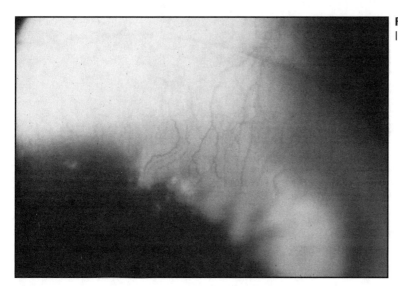

Figure 10-2. Neovascularization.

(with a minor thickening of the limbal tissue) and small, discrete corneal punctate staining or limbal infiltrates.

VLK: There is moderate to severe injection at the 3 to 9 o'clock positions adjacent to corneal staining and/or a dellen formation.

Treatment:

SLK is treated by discontinuing the use of solutions to which the patient may be hypersensitive. Substitute a non-preserved care product such as peroxide and encourage the use of lubricants. Consider frequent replacement daily wear lenses, either soft or rigid. If necessary, the underlying inflammation may be treated with a combination antibiotic/steroid.

VLK is treated by reducing lens wear time, increasing edge lift, reducing lens diameter, and encouraging the use of lubricant agents or vitamin A drops (for cellular rejuvenation). The underlying inflammation may be treated with a combination antibiotic/steroid.

Subepithelial Infiltrates

Definition: Subepithelial infiltrates (SEI) are an inflammatory reaction secondary to chronic hypoxia, causing a collection of cellular components (the infiltrate) just under the epithelium. SEI in the contact lens wearer can also be part of an immune response, solution reaction, mechanical irritation, or local infection.

Observation: The cornea becomes inflamed and white blood cells collect in discreet white-gray subepithelial pockets. A corneal scar may be confused for an infiltrate, neither of which stain with fluorescein.

Symptoms and Findings: The patient may have subtle symptoms ranging from mild to moderate. There may be discomfort, tearing, photophobia, decreased visual acuity, irritation, and/or a foreign body sensation.

Treatment: Contact lenses are discontinued until resolution. In most cases a hyperosmotic agent (such as 5% sodium chloride four times a day) or a steroid (such as fluorometholone if minor, soft steroids such as Vexol (Alcon Labs, Fort Worth, Tex) or Lotemax (Bausch & Lomb Pharmeceuticals, Rochester, NY), or prednisolone 1% if moderate to severe) is prescribed. The major concern is whether or not the infiltrate is actually a non-infectious sterile ulcer. In this case, a steroid would

Figure 10-3. Acute red eye with chemosis (conjunctival swelling).

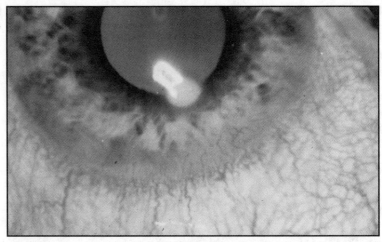

be contraindicated. (If there is a suspicion of ulcers, only an antibiotic is used.) The prognosis for SEI is highly favorable, with symptoms resolving in approximately 2 to 4 days. Infiltrates will resolve in 1 to 2 months. At that point, lens wear can be resumed.

Acute Red Eye

Definition: An acute red eye (ARE) is a sudden bulbar conjunctival response associated with either tight lens syndrome, dry eye, inflammatory reaction, mechanical irritation/abrasion, solulion toxemia, or hypersensitivity (Figure 10-3).

Observation: Redness is generally mild to moderate.

Symptoms and Findings: The patient may be somewhat uncomfortable and photophobic with blurred vision. The reaction may occur in one or both eyes.

Differential: Several contact lens-related and systemic differentials need to be considered such as keratitis, iritis, conjunctivitis (bacterial/viral/allergic), corneal abrasion or lesion, ulcer, SLK, VLK, and closed- or narrow-angle glaucoma.

Treatment: If the ARE is strictly associated with lens design, the redness will quickly resolve when the lens is removed without combined antibiotic/steroid therapy. This would imply that the lens is tight, which is causing conjunctival compression and congestion. A dry eye syndrome can easily be remedied with the use of wetting drops and/or punctal occlusion.

If the ARE is associated with a care product, the cornea will demonstrate some form of keratitis. This requires anti-inflammatory/antibiotic therapy and a different care product system. The patient should be re-educated on care product use and contact lens hygiene.

If an infection is suspected, cultures or microscope slides can be used to help decide which line of antibiotic therapy should be instituted. Cultures of the patient's storage case, solution vials, and contact lenses should also be obtained.

On resolution of the ARE, the soft lens patient can be refit to a daily wear lens of high Dk/L material with a moderate to high water content. Frequent replacement lenses should be considered (to maintain a higher level of hygiene). The storage case should be replaced periodically. The care system should be adjusted to include a more effective cleaning.

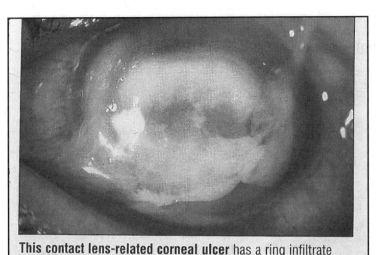

This contact lens-related corneal ulcer has a ring infiltrate and liquefactive necrosis of the corneal stroma.

Figure 10-4. Corneal ulcer.

Ulcerative Bacterial Keratitis Associated with Contact Lenses

Definition: A corneal ulcer is a form of a severe microbial infiltration of the corneal tissue (Figure 10-4). The ulcer will progressively destroy the underlying stroma, leading to possible perforation. Extended wear soft lenses have the greatest incidence of corneal ulcers. Patients who are immuno-compromised (ie, HIV, chemotherapy, or long-term steroid use), who have healing problems (such as diabetics), or who have severe dry eye may be more susceptible to either lens related or non-lens related ulcers. Table 10-1 shows the differential diagnosis of ulcerative keratitis versus subepithelial infiltrates.

The pathogens of concern are *Staphylococcus aureus* (gram-positive), *Staphylococcus epidermis* (gram-positive), *Pseudomonas aeruginosa* (gram-negative), *Streptococcus pneumoniae* (gram-negative), *Serratia marcescens* (gram-negative), *Acanthamoeba*, or fungi (*Candida, Aspergillus*). These are serious infections, and should be cared for by an eye practitioner.

Staphylococcal bacteria are usually transmitted by poor handling of contact lenses or contaminated solutions and/or cosmetic vials. It may also be associated with existing skin conditions. These ulcers demonstrate less severe subjective symptoms and objective findings.

Staphylococcal ulcers are usually associated with hypersensitivity caused by the waste products of the bacteria. This reaction can be noted around the periocular region (such as the lashes, conjunctival cul-de-sac, and nose). Staphylococcal ulcers have well-defined borders with a pale yellow coloration. They are similar to infiltrates in size, but are more dense. (It is often difficult to differentiate between a staph ulcer and an infiltrate.) The more severe ulcers tend to occur centrally. Marginal or paracentral peri-limbal ulcers are generally noninfectious, inflammatory reactions to by-products of the staph bacteria. Staphylococcal ulcers tend to not be as aggressive as Pseudomonas or other gram-negative ulcers.

Pseudomonas ulcers are usually associated with contaminated sources such as sinks, cosmetic or solution vials, and contact lens cases. These ulcers are more aggressive due to enzymes that contribute to the aggressive destruction of corneal tissue. A Pseudomonas ulcer can quickly progress to an abscess or perforation. In this case, it can "melt" the cornea within 24 to 48 hours if not properly treated.

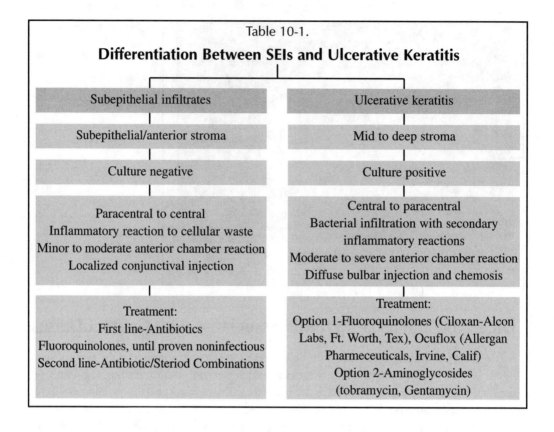

Table 10-1.
Differentiation Between SEIs and Ulcerative Keratitis

Subepithelial infiltrates	Ulcerative keratitis
Subepithelial/anterior stroma	Mid to deep stroma
Culture negative	Culture positive
Paracentral to central Inflammatory reaction to cellular waste Minor to moderate anterior chamber reaction Localized conjunctival injection	Central to paracentral Bacterial infiltration with secondary inflammatory reactions Moderate to severe anterior chamber reaction Diffuse bulbar injection and chemosis
Treatment: First line-Antibiotics Fluoroquinolones, until proven noninfectious Second line-Antibiotic/Steriod Combinations	Treatment: Option 1-Fluoroquinolones (Ciloxan-Alcon Labs, Ft. Worth, Tex), Ocuflox (Allergan Pharmeceuticals, Irvine, Calif) Option 2-Aminoglycosides (tobramycin, Gentamycin)

Pseudomonal ulcerations are centralized, amorphic (without a specific form), and dull in coloration, with a partial to moderately severe loss of corneal transparency. The organism generates large epithelial defects, dense stromal infiltrates, and edema. There is generally a significant anterior chamber reaction of cells, flare, and possibly hypopyon.

Observation: Conjunctival tissue will react in sympathy to the corneal response by exhibiting edema and increased injection (redness) around the limbus. Anterior chamber reactions may include cells, flare, and possibly hypopyon.

Symptoms and Findings: The patient will present with moderate to severe redness, pain, decreased vision, photophobia, discharge, and anterior chamber reaction (iritis or uveitis), generally in one eye only.

Treatment: The treatment of bacterial corneal ulcers depends on the causative organism. Staphylococcal ulcers are generally treated with fluoroquinolone or a combination antibiotic-steroid (such as tobramycin/dexamethosone or gentamicin/prednisolone). The aggressive Pseudomonas ulcer is also treated with fluoroquinolone. If the response of the anterior chamber is severe, the patient may be hospitalized and given intravenous antibiotic therapy.

Acanthamoeba Ulcers

Definition: *Acanthamoeba* is a free-living protozoan found in soil, sewage, tap water, well water, and sea water. It deserves a special mention here because *Acanthamoeba* can be present in improperly prepared homemade saline, which is used by some contact lens wearers. It can also live in a hot tub, infecting the unsuspecting contact lens wearer who does not remove his or her lenses before taking a dip.

Observation: The conjunctiva is red, there is profuse tearing, and the cornea will have punctate staining. There may be a corneal lesion that looks somewhat like a herpetic dendrite. The infection progresses to a severe inflammatory response, an anterior chamber reaction (including hypopyon), and a ring-shaped infiltration with recurrent epithelial breakdown and corneal decompensation leading to perforation.

Symptoms and Findings: The patient presents with ocular irritation, tearing, and discomfort or severe pain.

Treatment: Unfortunately, *Acanthamoeba* is highly resistant to antibiotic treatment. Treatment is very aggressive, and may include steroids, antibiotics, pupillary dilation, and other agents for approximately 2 months. In most cases the cornea cannot be saved. Scarring may be severe, later requiring a corneal graft.

Stromal Complications Secondary to Contact Lenses

Definition: When corneal edema occurs, fluid also leaks into the stromal layer. This may lead to striae or folds in the stroma, along with a central haze (Table 10-2).

Observation: Striae are fine, mesh-like, grayish-white vertical lines that do not interconnect. Folds are black, vertical, criss-crossing creases which represent a buckling of the cornea (Figure 10-5). Central corneal clouding appears as a whitened, bulging region throughout the stromal depth. The central clouding is evidence of severe epithelial thinning.

Symptoms and Findings: Patients will generally have no symptoms other than a minor to moderate level of lens awareness, glare sensitivity, and halos. Visual acuity will be slightly to moderately reduced. There may be some distortion noted when the eye is viewed with the keratometer.

Treatment: Lenses are discontinued until resolution. Hyperosmotic or steroid agents may be of assistance when there is appreciable cornea haze. If corneal edema is less than 5% (*caution level*), the patient requires a refit to high water content hydrogel or high Dk rigid gas permeable lenses on a daily wear schedule. If refitting to a hydrogel lens, it is adviseable to use a flatter BC to enhance lens movement and prevent lens stagnation on the eye. If the edema is between 5% to 8% (*danger level*) the same approach is used, favoring a high Dk rigid gas permeable lens. However, clinical aftercare and patient education needs to be more aggressive in order to monitor for more advanced signs of edema and possible corneal irregularities. Finally, if the edema exceeds 9% or greater (*pathological level*), lenses are discontinued and hypertonics are instituted. At this stage, corneal irregularities such as microcystic eruptions, a decrease in epithelial thickness, and an increase in stromal thickness will be noted. Lenses should not be refit until microcysts partially resolve and edema is reduced. When refitting, the patient should be limited strictly to daily wear, high Dk, or high water content lenses with adequate lens movement.

Endothelial Complications Secondary to Contact Lenses

Endothelial complications are the first signs of chronic hypoxia. Hypoxia degrades the integrity of the endothelial cells, leading to an imbalance in the normal equilibrium of oxygen and fluid. The effect can be transient, such as "blebs" and "bedewing," or more severe, observed as permanent changes in cell shape (polymegathism).

Table 10-2.
Corneal Edema Levels

Corneal Swelling	Signs	Relationships	Level
< 2%	Undetectable edema	Unknown	Benign
2% to 5%	Early stages of striae	Implies chronic hypoxia	Safe
5%	Vertical striae observed	Chronic hypoxia	Caution
8%	Posterior folds and striae	Acute edema	Danger
20%	Loss of comeal transparency, folds, striae	Pathological	Pathological

Adapted from Grant TJ, Terry R, Holden BA. Extended wear of hydrogel lenses: clinical problems and their management. In: London R, ed. Problems in Optometry: Contact Lenses and Ocular Disease. *Philadelphia, Pa: JB Lippincott Co;1990.*

Figure 10-5. Corneal folds.

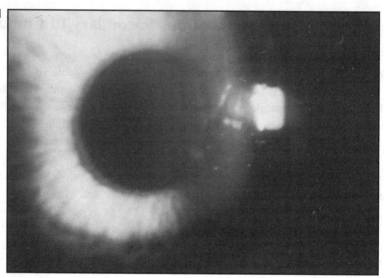

Endothelial Bedewing

Definition: Endothelial bedewing is an inflammatory response of the anterior uvea associated with micro-trauma.

Observation: Edematous droplets form on the posterior surface of the corneal endothelium. These are best visualized on high magnification with retroillumination

Symptoms and Treatment: Patients will be asymptomatic. No treatment is required.

Endothelial Blebs

Definition: Endothelial blebs are related to the sudden shock of contact lenses being introduced to the eye. This disturbs the endothelium and its normal fluid balance.[5] Blebs occur within the first 20 to 45 minutes after lens insertion and peak 20 to 30 minutes after appearing. The response indicates that the patient may not be a suitable extended wear candidate.

Observation: Large, apparent black holes in the endothelium.

Symptoms and Treatment: There are no symptoms. No treatment is required.

Endothelial Polymegathism and Pleomorphism

Definitions: These are long-term changes to endothelial cell shape and dimension due to age and/or hypoxia. Polymegathism (literally, "many oversized") is a change in cell size leading to deformity. Pleomorphism (literally, "more forms") is a change in the normal hexagonal symmetry of the endothelial cells. Stress on the cornea, such as contact lenses, diabetes, glaucoma, acute or recurrent anterior uveitis, trauma, or cataract extraction (or other intraocular surgical procedures), can induce these changes. Polymegathism is a permanent change to the cell structure that can indicate future corneal compromise, particularly during invasive, intraocular surgical procedures.

Symptoms and Findings: The patient will be asymptomatic.

Observations: There will be an increase in cell size variation, a decrease in the endothelial cell density, and a decrease in the continuity of the endothelial mosaic structure. These changes are best observed via specular microscopy.

Treatment: Since the cellular changes are due to oxygen flow, the patient should be refit with daily wear high water content soft or high Dk rigid lenses. The goal of therapy is to reduce corneal stress and enhance oxygen transport.

Staining Patterns

Tight Lens Syndrome or Immobile Lens Syndrome

Definition: Tight or immobile lens syndrome is a lens fitting relationship that is unacceptably steep.

Observation: When stained with fluorescein, the examiner will note a ring of stain caused by compression around the central cornea (rigid lenses) or limbus (hydrogel) (Figure 10-6), with conjunctival redness at the limbus. The lens will be decentered inferiorly and somewhat immobile even with a strong, forced blink. Minimal fluorescein will be seen underneath the lens, while an excessive amount will pool at the lens edge.

Symptoms and Findings: The patient will complain that the lenses are difficult to remove. The visual acuity may be variable, or there may be visual blur after removing the lenses. In addition, once the lenses are removed, the patient will have the urge to rub the eyes vigorously.

Treatment: There may be severe induced punctate keratopathy with corneal distortion and edema that may require prophylactic antibiotics and/or combination antibiotic/steroid therapy. If the cornea is clear, refit the patient with a flatter BC and/or a smaller optic zone while encouraging the use of wetting drops, particularly prior to lens removal.

3-9 Staining

Definition: 3-9 staining is associated with a rigid lens where the edge is excessively sharp or poorly rounded. Thirty percent of rigid gas permeable lens wearers will have some level of 3-9 staining.

Observations and Symptoms: A patch punctate keratopathy appears near the limbus. 3-9 staining can be graded as follows: Stage 1 has small, discrete punctate staining with no symptoms. Stage 2 demonstrates a mild level of patch superficial punctate keratitis (SPK). Stage 3 demonstrates a dense patch keratopathy and adjacent conjunctival injection or vascularization with a significant decrease in wear time tolerance. In Stage 4 there is a dellen, with lens intolerance and a significantly increased in limbal vascular response.

Figure 10-6. Conjunctival impression ring.

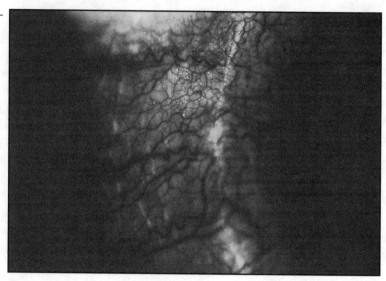

Treatment: In Stage 3 or 4, the acute inflammatory reaction is treated with a combination antibiotic/steroid therapy. It is appropriate to increase axial edge lift and to round the lens edges with a smooth blend (see Chapter 9). Lenses should be stored in solution rather than dry. In addition, rewetting drops should be used frequently during wear.

Corneal Dellen

Definition: Dellen (small, concave structures) form as a result of accumulated dried-out epithelium, associated with prolonged chafing of the epithelium by a rigid lens. Dellen are the final result of long-term 3-9 staining.

Observation: Dellen have variable density and loss of corneal translucency (Figure 10-7). They can be mistaken for a marginal ulcer.

Treatment: Reduce lens wear time, increase edge lift, encourage the use of lubricant agents or vitamin A (for cellular rejuvenation), reduce lens diameter. If necessary, the underlying inflammation may be treated with a combination antibiotic/steroid therapy.[6]

Superficial Punctate Keratitis

`OptT`

Definition: SPK has multiple causes and variable patterns (Figure 10-8). The term is really a "catch-all" phrase implying that there is an epithelial inflammation secondary to insult. In the contact lens wearer, the insult could be from infection, allergy, micro-trauma, mechanical abrasion, hypoxia, solution toxemia, or lens-induced dryness.

Observations: SPK stains as small spots, often in the center or just slightly below (see Figure 10-8). There may be a few here and there, or they may be localized in a dense grouping.

Symptoms and Findings: The patient might notice mild to moderate changes in acuity, a foreign body sensation, changes in lens awareness, and an increase in corneal sensitivity.

Treatment: SPK treatment protocol depends on the underlying cause. If the cause is not lens associated, a culture and subsequent antibiotic and/or steroid therapy should be instituted. If the SPK *is* lens related, lens use should be discontinued immediately and antibiotic and/or steroid therapy started.

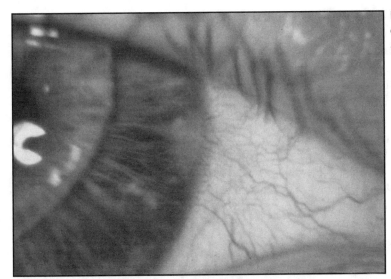

Figure 10-7. Corneal dellen (rigid gas permeable lens related).

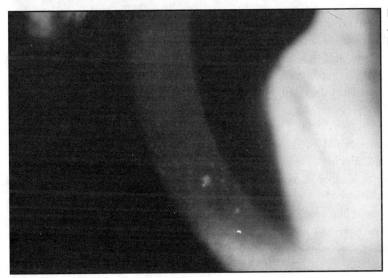

Figure 10-8. Discrete and diffuse superficial keratitis.

After the SPK has cleared, monitor for recurrent corneal erosion syndrome or dry eye. If the patient is to be refit with contact lenses, a low water content disposable or frequent replacement daily wear lens with use of rewetting drops is advised. Also tell the patient about environmental factors that may effect lens wear, such as poor ventilation, low humidity, alcohol consumption, and diuretics.

Dehydration Keratitis

OptT

Definition: Dehydration keratitis is due to poor hydrogel lens wetting, which leads to steepening and vaulting of the lens away from the corneal surface. As the lens vaults, an air pocket replaces the normal tear film, leaving the superficial epithelium to dry and chafe with each movement of the lens. The problem usually has a higher association with extended wear versus daily wear hydrogels.

Observation: The staining is usually an inferior, arched, coalesced band of punctate staining with epithelial thickening.

Symptoms and Findings: The patient will have a mild to moderate level of lens awareness, a decreased wearing time, mild ocular redness, increased burning or foreign body sensation, and an increased need for wetting drops. There is also a decrease in both visual quality and acuity, particularly with toric and bifocal soft contacts.

Treatment: Antibiotics are used to prevent infection for 24 to 48 hours until resolution of epithelial staining. Lens wear can be resumed after a detailed tear film analysis. If the tear film is sufficient to handle the lens, a low water content, frequent replacement lens of a slightly greater center thickness should be used. (Low water content, slightly thicker lenses will tend to retain their properties longer than a thin, high water content lens.) Lubricant therapy should be instituted as well as punctal occlusion if deemed necessary.

Solution Toxemia

Definition: Solution toxemia is an acute keratitis caused by a hypersensitivity reaction to a care product. The reaction can be allergic in nature or induced by a chemical burn (ie, peroxide or daily cleaner). An acute hypersensitivity reaction to a chemical insult is commonly associated with thimerosal, chlorohexidine, or benzalkonium chloride preservatives.

Observation: There will be mild to severe bulbar redness, swelling, diffuse SPK, and increased dilation of the blood vessels surrounding the limbus.

Symptoms and Findings: The patient will immediately complain of an acute itchy or gritty sensation, mild to severe photophobia, redness, discomfort to pain, decrease in vision, and a watery discharge.

Treatment: The clinician should investigate the history of care product use. If the solution toxemia is contact lens related, it is important to identify if the problem is a delayed hypersensitivity to a care product ingredient, such as thimerosal, or if it is an acute reaction to exposure, as with peroxide misuse. If it is a delayed hypersensitivity, the eye may be treated with a mild steroid. If it is an acute exposure, treat it like a sudden chemical exposure. On resolution of the keratopathy, re-educate patient about care product procedures, emphasizing proper neutralization and rinsing as well as lens replacement. You might consider a new care system such as a preservative-free product.

OptT

Corneal Abrasions and Foreign Body Tracking

Definition: Corneal abrasions and foreign body tracking is the chafing or drying of the epithelium created by lens fracture or defect, lens deposits, foreign bodies, or blunt trauma as demonstrated by a distinct path or pattern of corneal staining (Table 10-3).

Observations: A corneal abrasion is localized and deep, with a spread of fluorescein within the defect. Foreign body tracking is more superficial (Figure 10-9). If either the abrasion or tracking is related directly to the lens, the lens should be inspected for defects. In most cases, the epithelial defect will mimic the size and shape of the lens defect.

Symptoms and Findings: The patient may present with a variety of symptoms and signs, including a sudden onset of discomfort or pain, a sandy or gritty sensation, mild to moderate redness, excessive tearing, and lid edema and swelling. The response may be immediate if an abrasion is created on insertion. The response may be delayed if the lens is shielding the cornea from atmospheric exposure.

Table 10-3. Grading Scale for Epithelial Staining		
Grade	**Extent**	**Depth**
O (None)	Absent	Absent
1 (Trace)	1% to 15% surface involvement	Superficial epithelial
2 (Mild)	16% to 30% surface involvement	Stromal glow within 30 seconds after NaFI instillation
3 (Moderate)	31% to 45% surface involvement	Immediate, localized stromal glow
4 (Severe)	46% or greater surface involvement	Immediate, diffuse stromal glow

Adapted from Grant TJ, Terry R. Holden BA. Soft lens extended wear. In: Harris MG, ed. Contact Lenses: Treatment Options for Ocular Disease. *New York, NY: Mosby Publishing; 1996.*

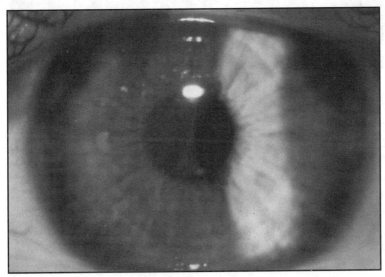

Figure 10-9. Foriegn body tracking.

Treatment: In any of these situations, contact lens wear should be discontinued. Treatment for an abrasion is much more aggressive than for a foreign body track. Because the epithelium is broken in either case, antibiotics are often given as a preventative against infection. After instillation of antibiotic ointment the eye may be lightly patched. (Ointments are preferred over drops secondary to their lubricating effect.)

Contact Lens Induced Papillary Conjunctivitis, or Giant Papillary Conjunctivitis

OptT

Definition: Giant Papillary Conjunctivitis (GPC) received its name from Allansmith (et al.) who described the palpebral conjunctival lid formations as elevations with central vascularization (Figure 10-10). These are different from follicles, which are fluid-filled and do not have a blood vessel in the center. GPC in contact lens wearers is generally considered to be caused by an allergic reaction to surface deposits and/or constant mechanical irritation of the palpebral conjunctiva by the contact lens.

Observations: In GPC, the surface of the palpebral conjunctiva (notably the upper lid) is covered with papillae. The papillae vary in size from 0.5 mm and greater. With the instillation of flu-

Figure 10-10. Contact induced papillary conjunctivitis.

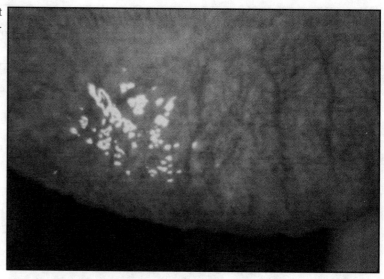

orescein, distinct crevices can be visualized between each papilla. GPC is best observed using white, diffuse light on low magnification.

The papillae tend to grab the contact lens on the blink and hold it in a slightly superior decentered position, while impeding the downward movement of the lens. Due to the constant irritation of the palpebral conjunctiva, a reactive mucus discharge occurs, leading to additional deposits on the lens surface.

Symptoms and Findings: GPC can be graded into four levels of severity.[7] Stage 1 demonstrates no anatomical signs and only minor symptoms of mucus discharge and itching. Stage 2 exhibits papillary enlargement to 0.5 mm (but less than 1.0 mm), mucus strands, redness, and an increase in lens deposits. The patient will describe itchiness, discharge, lens awareness, and blurred acuity. Stage 3 shows papillae greater than 1.0 mm and increased mucus, lens awareness, and redness. There will also be edema and lens decentration superiorly. The patient will describe moderate to severe symptoms with decreased wear time, frequent lens depositing, and increased lens movement and blur. Stage 4 demonstrates papillae larger than 1.0 mm which have a mushroom shape, accompanied by severe symptoms and signs.

Treatment: Stage 1 requires no intervention other than refitting with a frequent replacement or disposable lens. Another option would be to continue conventional lenses using a peroxide care product with enzyme cleaning.

Stage 2 requires lens replacement, frequent irrigation with lubricating drops to reduce mucus, and possibly a prescription for a mast cell stabilizer.

Stage 3 requires discontinuation of lenses for a short time and use of a mast cell stabilizer or low concentration steroid. Lenses can be refit to disposable or frequent replacement lenses with peroxide care products until resolution of the papillae.

Stage 4 requires complete discontinuation of lenses as well as use of steroids, both until resolution. Upon resolution, frequent replacement or disposable lenses should be fit using a peroxide care system.

References

1. Weissman BA, Mondino B. Corneal ulcers associated with extended wear soft contact lenses. *Am J Ophthalmol.* 1984;97:476-481.

2. Jantzi ID, et al. Corneal vascularization in a group of soft contact wearers: prevalence, magnitude, type, and related factors. *Canadian Journal of Optometry.* 1987;49:174.

3. Depaolis MD, Shovlin JP. Contact lenses and anterior segment disease: considerations in differential diagnosis. *Practical Optometry.* 1993;4(4):142-146.

4. Fuerst DJ, Sugar J, Worobec S. Superior limbic keratoconjunctivitis associated with contact lens wearers. *Ophthalmology.* 1983;90:616.

5. Vannas A, Makitie J, Sulonen J. Contact lens induced transient changes to the endothelium. *Acta Ophthalmol.* 1981;59:552-559.

6. Lebow KA. Peripheral corneal staining. In: Silbert JA, ed. *Anterior Segment Complications of Contact Lens Wear.* New York, NY: Churchill Livingstone; 1994.

7. Allansmith MR. Giant papillary conjunctivitis. *J Am Optom Assoc.* 1990;61(suppl):S42.

Chapter 11

Contact Lenses for Presbyopes

KEY POINTS

- Patient selection is based on motivation, realistic expectations, and the ability to accept minor visual compromise.

- When refining monovision, leave the patient with a subtle blur of approximately 20/25 at distance and near.

- Multifocal contact lenses can be described as "simultaneous view designs" due to their position over the pupil.

- The annular or concentric design multifocal lens utilizes a center/near (periphery/distance) or center/distance (periphery/near) design.

- Aspheric multifocals utilize a pseudo-annular design and are generally referred to as progressive power lenses.

- Translating or alternating bifocal lens designs are essentially "miniature" executive, flat top, or crescent style bifocals that are position-dependent.

- The patient should be educated that a translating lens design will be "low riding," which can cause easier dislodgment and loss of the lens.

Introduction

Presbyopia is defined as the decrease in accommodative ability that occurs with aging. Plus power is required to compensate for the inability to focus at a near working distance.

The success of presbyopic fitting depends on many factors. The primary factor is motivation. Contact lenses for presbyopia must not be presented as a "cure-all," but as an alternative with some compromises to vision.

Patient selection is premised by age and refraction. The younger presbyope will adapt to a presbyopic contact lens correction more easily than an older patient will. Likewise, a patient requiring a lower add power will also be more accepting of a presbyopic contact lens correction than a patient requiring a higher add power. Finally, hyperopes tend to be the best candidates. Emmetropes are generally the least accepting of the visual compromise induced by presbyopic corrections.

In all forms of presbyopic fitting, the dominant eye will need to be selected in order to bias one eye for distance and the other for near (Table 11-1). The easiest way to do this is as follows:

1) The patient is asked to fully extend the arms, placing the hands together to make a "frame" (about the size of a quarter) with the thumbs and index fingers.

2) The patient is asked to keep both eyes opened and target an isolated letter on the acuity chart through the frame.

3) The patient keeps the arms and hands up, framing the letter, while the fitter covers one eye and then the other.

4) The eye that sees the target through the frame is the dominant eye.

Lens Design Options

There are many lens designs available, each having a different level of complexity in fitting and ability to satisfy the visual and environmental needs of the patient. The designs include monovision, modified monovision, simultaneous view bifocals, and translating bifocals (Table 11-2).

Monovision

Monovision utilizes the patient's present single vision contact lens design with a subtle power adjustment to bias one eye to near and the other to distance. The early presbyope will have a higher success rate in being fit with monovision due to a lesser add power requirement and thus a lesser visual compromise.

Patient selection is based on the need for nearpoint correction. If monovision is introduced too soon, the patient will not be able to adapt visually. The patient must have a nearpoint visual complaint and/or accept a minimum of a +1.00 add. A +1.00 spectacle add will translate to a +0.75 contact lens add, leaving the patient with a subtle blur of approximately 20/25 at distance and near. (A lesser add is used with monovision in order to minimize near and distance disparity.)

When refining a monovision correction, the near eye should be able to achieve a distance visual acuity of approximately 20/40 to 20/50 vision (Table 11-3). This level is critical in operating a motor vehicle.

Refinement of monovision should start with the addition of plus to the distance eye. If the patient accepts additional plus in the distance eye without affecting distance acuity, it will enhance near and intermediate ranges. Next, try additional plus in the near eye while the patient looks at the distant chart. Again, if distance vision is not diminished, this will be a benefit for close range work. If additional power, plus or minus, does not improve the quality of vision, the fitter can suggest some other contact lens option.

OptA

Table 11-1.

Determination of the Distance Dominant Eye

Method	Technique
Hole in the hand (Demonstrates visual dominance and alignment)	1. The patient is asked to fully extend the arms and place the hands together, making an opening the approximate size of a quarter. 2. The patient is asked to view an isolated letter on the acuity chart through the opening. 3. The fitter then covers one eye and then the other 4. The eye that sees the target through the "hole" is the dominant eye.
Plus lens test (Demonstrates ocular dominance and level of "blur toleration")	1. Place the best distance refraction into a trial fume. 2. Place a +1.50 lens in front of each eye in an alternating fashion as the patient views the distance acuity chart. Note: The test should be performed with an add power +0.25 to +0.50 less than the patient's spectacle add. 3. Ask the patient: "When the lens is held over your eye, which eye is least disturbed or appreciates the least amount of blur?" 4. The eye which appreciates the least amount of blur is the eye which should be selected for distance dominance. (Less add power is required due to the vertex effect. Closer to the corneal plane adds plus to the overall power.)
Alternate occlusion (Demonstrates the dominant eye for distance visual)	1. This method uses a "cover test" method to determine the distance dominant eye. 2. Simply have the patient view the distance acuity chart while occluding the eyes in an alternating format. 3. Ask the patient which eye appreciates the sharpest quality of vision while alternating the occluder. The eye with the sharpest vision is the dominant eye. 4. After determining the distance dominant eye in this method, proceed to the "plus lens" method to determine the level of "blur tolerance" at distance and near.
"Camera to the eye" or "Targeting eye" method (Defines distance dominant eye)	1. Place the final distance correction into a trial frame. 2. Have the patient take a camera and put it to the eye they would normally use to take pictures. This is their dominant distance eye. 3. If a patient is active in sports which require firearms, archery, and so forth, ask the patient which eye they would usually use for targeting. Again this would be the dominant distance eye. 4. After the dominant eye is determined, proceed with the introduction of plus lenses over the near eye to determine the tolerance for blur.
Refractive Variance	Generally, the more myopic (or least hyperopic) eye will accept less plus at near point. Therefore, the more myopic eye should be biased for the distance correction.

The limitations of monovision occur particularly in dim lighting situations such as driving at night or during sports activities. The patient should be given an option to utilize a third, spare distance contact lens to be used instead of the near contact when performing "distance only" tasks.

A second alternative for visual enhancement with monovision is a spectacle overcorrection. A nearpoint overcorrection should have a suitable add power to assist the farpoint biased eye. Ideally, if the spectacle overcorrection is required for distance, the lens should be prescribed as a photosensitive or clip-on sunglass lens.

Table 11-2.
Contact Lens Options for Presbyopes

✔ = below average   ✔✔ = average   ✔✔✔ = above average

Factor	Monovision	Modified Monovision	Translating Bifocal	Simultaneous Design	Modified Bivision
Visual demand at distance	✔✔	✔✔✔	✔✔✔	✔✔	✔✔✔
Visual demands at intermediate	✔	✔✔	✔	✔✔✔	✔✔✔
Visual demands at nearpoint	✔✔	✔✔	✔✔✔	✔✔	✔✔✔
Add power	< +1.75	< +2.50	< +2.50	< +1.75	< +2.50
Pupil dependency	none	minimal	variable	variable	variable
Pupil size limitations (mm)	no limitation	> 3	3 to 4	3 to 4	3 to 4
Expense	low to moderate	average to moderate	high	variable	high

All modalities are available in rigid lens materials in various designs. Hydrogel lenses are available in the various designs with a more limited, but expanding, availability.

Table 11-3.

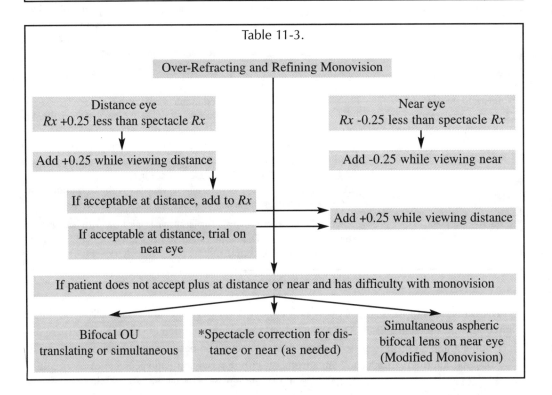

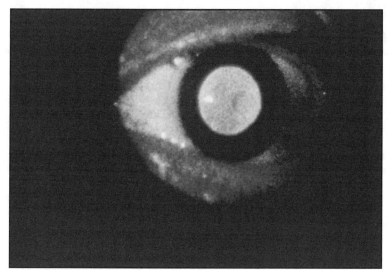

Figure 11-1. Alges annular soft bifocal (Unilens, Largo, Fla).

Simultaneous View Annular Bifocals

Multifocal contact lenses can be described as simultaneous view designs due to their position over the pupil (Figure 11-1). The lens has to be properly centered over the pupil and visual axis to yield the optimal visual effect. Any decentration will degrade the visual quality. Lens centration can be improved by utilizing a steeper BC as long as it maintains the proper ocular physiological balance.

The annular or concentric design multifocal lens utilizes a center/near (periphery/distance) or center/distance (periphery/near) design. Center/near designs are used to maximize vision in variable lighting conditions when the pupil is mid-dilated. In contrast, center/distance designs are used to maximize the optics in better lighting conditions. The main disadvantage of concentric lenses is the induced blur circle created by the lens optics.

The major limitation to the center/distance design is that room lighting in normal working conditions limits the functional nearpoint of the lens. In order to combat this problem, one could use either different segment sizes on each eye or inverse designs. For example, the right eye could be fit with a center/near design and the left fit with a center/distance design. The power would be biased such that the one eye would facilitate near and intermediate while the dominant eye would be biased to intermediate and distance.

Simultaneous View Aspheric and Multi-Zonal Multifocals

Aspheric multifocal designs utilize a pseudo-annular design that is generally referred to as a progressive power design. Simultaneous view aspheric multifocals have the advantage of allowing for a wide range of correctable vision at near, intermediate, and distance without adjusting the head or eye position.

Aspheric lens designs require the fitter to bias one eye to distance (infinity) and 25 to 35 inches (intermediate), and the other eye to 18 to 24 inches (proximal intermediate) and 14 to 18 inches (near).[1,2,3,4] In addition, aspheric lenses are pupil and visual axis-dependent.

There are various aspheric lens designs. The success rate can be enhanced by abiding to the key principles of pupil and visual axis centration, adjusting powers to meet the patient's needs, and selecting the appropriate material to meet the eye's physiological requirements.

Aspheric multifocal designs are based on e value. (When referring to contact lenses, the term eccentricity refers to the progressive flattening of the lens surface, from the center to the periphery. The e value will be zero for a sphere and approach the value of 1 for a parabola. The degree of flattening is directly proportional to the increase in the eccentricity.)

In non-presbyopic lenses, aspherics are used to complement the topography of the cornea. The e value of the cornea will be about 0.3 or spherical. However, flatter keratometric values will demonstrate an e value around 0.7 or approaching a parabolic contour. For example, when low eccentricity lenses are fit on the cornea, a marked clearance will appear in the fluorescein pattern.

Front surface aspherics are generally used for presbyopic correction. The amount of add required for an aspheric lens will also require an e value of 1 to 1.3. A value of 1 would be analogous to a low add, such as +1.00, and a value of 1.3 would be equivalent to a +2.50 add. (e values of 0.4 to 0.6 are usually prescribed for non-presbyopic patients and are used to enhance the fitting characteristics of the lens.)[5,6]

Explain to the patient that there will be some compromise in the quality of vision, but that there will be an enhanced level of vision at various ranges. There is no one design that will meet the total visual needs of the patient, therefore combinations of powers and designs must be tried. Follow the specific guidelines developed by each manufacturer for the initial trial fitting and then apply creativity and clinical experience to determine the appropriate refinement.

Translating or Alternating Bifocal Lens Designs

Translating or alternating bifocal lens designs are essentially "miniature" executive, straight top (ST), or crescent style bifocals that are pupil-dependent (Figures 11-2, 3, and 4). All light will pass through the distance or near zone based on the position of the eye and the lens.

Hydrophilic translating designs have not proven to be effective due to the lack of significant position alternation between distance and near. Rigid translating bifocals can be fabricated in front, back, and bitoric designs. Translating bifocal lenses, particularly single piece lenses, are 30% to 40% thicker than standard rigid spherical lenses. Ideally, the patient should have experience with rigid lenses prior to fitting rigid translating bifocals.

The basic fitting of these lenses does not vary significantly from standard gas permeable techniques. Prior to fitting, pupil size in bright, moderate, and dim light must be measured. Large pupil diameters will limit the success of a crescent or segmented bifocal. Palpebral aperture width and lid tension will also have a significant effect on lens fitting. Tight lids will not allow the lens to translate properly and also may displace the bifocal segment superiorly. Flaccid lids will allow the lens to displace inferiorly.

The lens will assume an inferior position in primary distance gaze. To ensure this position, the lens requires stabilization (ballasting and truncation similar to toric lenses). These lenses require a palpebral aperture or inferior aperture position. An experienced rigid lens patient who will be refit with a translating design should be forewarned that the lens position will be low in comparison to the previous lens.

The optimal fitting scenario for a translating bifocal is to position the segment line below the pupillary fringe at mid-dilation. (The segment height will vary based on lens design.) Observe the segment position in primary gaze, then have the patient look slightly down and inward while you observe the translation of the segment. This is best accomplished by using a cobalt blue filter with the slit lamp on a moderate to low illumination. The segment should never position itself within the pupil on distance gaze, but should have a complete coverage of the pupil on near gaze.

Translating lenses should be fit with an alignment fit to slightly steeper than the flattest K.

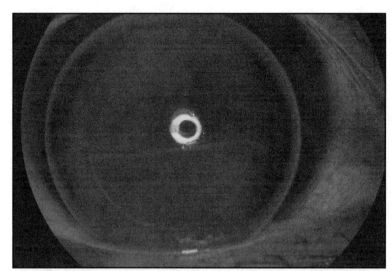

Figure 11-2. Paragon ST (Paragon, Mesa, Ariz).

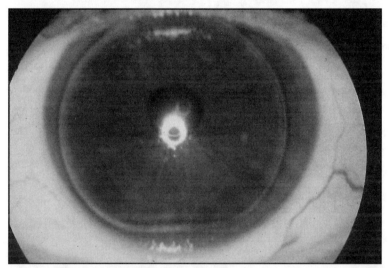

Figure 11-3. Optimal position for the Paragon ST translating bifocal.

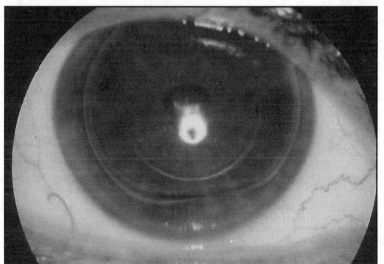

Figure 11-4. Superior displacement of the Paragon ST.

To compensate for excessive steepness, an optic zone equal to or slightly smaller than the BC should be used. Additionally, the fitter should incorporate the appropriate prism ballast to allow the lens to settle evenly on the inferior lid margin. The prism ballast for a minus lens will be 2 to 2.5 diopters, while a plus lens will require 1.5 to 2 diopters. To enhance the prism ballast and reduce overall lens thickness, a truncation can be added. Truncation should range up to 0.4 mm; 0.2 mm is usually sufficient.

Rotation of a translating lens is considered problematic if the segment encroaches into part of the pupil or is excessively nasal or temporal. Lens rotation can be corrected by specifying the base apex line. This is done in the same manner as adjusting for a toric rotation, using the LARS principle.

To avoid superior lid attachment, the PCR system can be designed steeper than normal. Additionally, a superior CN bevel or superior tapering of the front surface will limit superior lid grab.

References

1. Lapierre M, et al. Success rate evaluation of simultaneous center add soft contact lenses. *International Contact Lens Clinic*. 1989;19(3):157-161.

2. Shapiro MB, Bredeson DC. A prospective evaluation of Unilens soft multifocal contact lens in 100 patients. *CLAO*. July 1994;20(3):189-191.

3. Key JE, Morris K, Mobley C. Perspective clinical evaluation of the Sunsoft multifocal contact lens. *CLAO*. July 1996;22(3):179-184.

4. Maltzman BA, Harris M, Espy J. Experience with soft bifocal contact lenses. *CLAO*. 1985;11:73-77.

5. Baude D, Meige C. Presbyopia with contact lenses—a new aspherical progressive lens. *British Contact Lens Association*. 1992;15(1):7-15.

6. Goldberg IB. Basic principles of aspheric contact lenses. *Contact Lens Forum*. May 1998;35-38.

Chapter 12

Special Topics

KEY POINTS

- The primary indication for contact lens wear in infants is following unilateral or bilateral cataract extraction.

- The infant or small child must become comfortable working around the eyes. This is accomplished by a gentle facial and eyelid massage by the parent and the clinician.

- Aphakic lenses are high plus with an increased mass and highly convex anterior front curve. These features may lead to handling and physiological difficulties.

- Aphakic rigid lens power is best determined using a manifest refraction in conjunction with a diagnostic lens over-refraction with vertex compensation.

- After refractive surgery, the flattened corneal cap will cause a biconvex lens (plus lens) effect, yielding a minus over-refraction.

- Hydrogel bandage lenses provide an increase in surface wetting, foster a more regular refracting surface, reduce exposure sensitivity, assist in wound healing, and splint corneal defects.

- Contact lenses for keratoconus should contour the corneal shape, yielding a balance of bearing and clearance across the corneal surface.

Pediatric Contact Lens Fitting

A successful pediatric contact lens candidate is one who is able to physiologically tolerate a contact lens, while benefiting visually. In addition, the adult caregiver must accept responsibility for handling both lenses and follow-up. Indications for the use of contact lenses in those under 5 years of age involve high refractive errors, aphakia, irregular astigmatism, and aniseikonia. Spectacles can be used in many of these cases except congenital aphakia, where contact lenses are preferred.

Pediatric Aphakia

The primary indication for contact lens wear in infants is following unilateral or bilateral cataract extraction. Spectacles are usually the first choice, particularly in cases of bilateral aphakia. Intraocular lenses are not recommended for this age group.

Contact lenses offer several advantages and disadvantages in aphakia. The major advantage is that the optical correction can be easily changed to correspond to ocular growth without additional surgery. The contact lens also allows for an optimal refractive correction at the corneal ' plane, thus minimizing aniseikonia and encouraging visual development. Difficulties include lens care, maintenance, and handling, which must be performed by parents or guardians. In addition, there may be some initial discomfort for the patient.

Aphakic infants are usually fit with flexible silicone lenses (Table 12-1). Advantages of these lenses include increased corneal oxygenation and lens comfort. Disadvantages include the cost of the lens, inability to obtain full optical correction (due to limited parameters), rapid soilage of the lens, and occasional corneal abrasion.

Hydrogel lenses are the preferred modality for pediatric aphakic correction, if lens parameters are available.[1] This modality affords the patient enhanced comfort, as well as easy insertion and removal. Disadvantages of a hydrogel lens include fragility, poor correction of residual astigmatism, and frequent lens loss (in some).

Flexible wear, or limiting the amount of nocturnal lens wear, is the preferable schedule for patient comfort and parent convenience. This schedule also limits the potential for adverse reactions associated with extended wear.

Lens power is determined by objective refraction via retinoscopy (which will need to be vertex corrected). Secondly, keratometry or corneal topography should be obtained to determine corneal curvature values. However, such measurements may be extremely difficult with infants. In this case, the fitter must guess at the BC and use a trial lens.

Material Selection and Fitting Characteristics

Lens selection should be based on the visual and physiological requirements of the patient with respect to the ease and economics of lens replacement. Lens materials should incorporate an ultravliolet (UV) blocking agent if available. Rigid gas permeables with a high Dk can be used, however, the initial lenses of choice are usually the Silsoft lens (Bausch & Lomb, Claremont, Calif) or soft contact lenses, preferably extended wear.

Silicone lenses are fit using an "on K" philosophy. A 7.5 mm BC is the first lens to be evaluated if the child is less than 2 years of age. A 7.7 mm BC is chosen for children between 2 and 4 years of age, and 7.9 mm BC if the child is older than 4 years. Fluorescein should demonstrate a light apical touch. A diameter of 11.3 mm is selected first. (The lens diameter is limited to

Table 12-1.
Advantages and Disadvantages of Extended Wear Silicone Contact Lenses

Advantages:

Greatest flow of oxygen of any material available today
Increased thermal conductivity
Stability of power
Lack of bacterial contamination
Decreased loss rate over conventional lenses
Better acuity than hydrogel lens
Comfort
Easy to fit

Disadvantages:

Mucus and lipid build-up on posterior surface
Breakdown of hydrophilic surface
One lens diameter for pediatric aphakia

Adapted from Rogers GL. Extended wear silicone contact lenses in children with cataracts. Ophthalmology. *1980;87:867.*

11.3 mm for the pediatric design.) Fitting the silicone lens requires little cooperation from the patient. Keratometric readings are unnecessary. An initial trial lens is selected on the assumption that the youngest children have the steepest corneas.

Rigid lenses should also be fit "on K" with slightly smaller overall diameters. Lens diameter should be selected based on the orbital and ocular size of the patient. Additionally, power corrections for nearpoint viewing will need to be incorporated, around +3.00 for the infant. The optic zone should be equal to or slightly greater than the BC (in millimeters). It is also advisable to lenticulate the lens for proper centration and lens movement. If a lens is fit "on K" and the optic zone and subsequent lens diameter are large, the lens will vault the cornea and show central fluorescein pooling with restricted tear exchange and movement. Smaller lenses will move excessively and tend to decenter.

Fitting Techniques

The infant or small child must become comfortable with someone working around his or her eyes. This is accomplished by a gentle facial and eyelid massage by the parent and the clinician.

The easiest position for lens insertion on an infant is to have the child lie on the parent's lap along the adult's thigh. The feet of the child should be toward the parent, and the head positioned towards the clinician. It is helpful to immobilize the child by wrapping him or her comfortably in a blanket or sheet. This will prevent erratic movement.

Inserting a contact lens requires the retraction of the child's eyelids by the clinician, assistant, or parent. (This becomes difficult if the child is crying. Place a drop of anesthetic onto the lens as a wetting agent.) Grasp the lens by pinching the lens edge between the thumb and forefinger so that it fans outward. Using the middle finger on the same hand with the lens, retract the lower lid. Using the opposite hand, massage the upper lid and then retract. Place the opened end of the lens under the upper lid onto the superior conjunctiva and then lower the lens onto the superior cornea. The lens will center after lid closure. Immediately after insertion the parent is encouraged to cradle and comfort the child. Allow the child to relax prior to examination of the lens.

Lens removal is performed in the same manner. Retract the superior lid by resting your thumb on the child's head and grasp the upper lid with the forefinger. The lower lid is retracted by pulling the lid downward with the middle finger and pinching the lens at 6 o'clock below the limbus. Grasp the lens and quickly remove it with care not to tear the lens. (If the lens should tear, inspect the eye, particularly under the lid, for any missing section of the lens. A drop of anesthetic may be beneficial.)

The parent must also be taught these techniques. Once the child has experienced it several times, he or she will not be as combative.

Contact Lens Parameters

Power

Power is best determined via objective retinoscopy. If the clinician is not able to obtain a reasonable retinoscopic result, one can predict the power needs by calculating the corneal curvature and axial length obtained through ultrasound. Power changes over time can be predicted and need to be addressed frequently. A high plus power is expected to decrease approximately 10 D over the first 11 to 18 months of life. The mean spherical equivalent changes from +31.16 D at 1 month to only +18.99 D at 48 months.

Corneal Curvature and Base Curve

The corneal curvature of an infant or pediatric patient is difficult to obtain. Therefore, one must depend on automation or clinical study results. Studies have indicated that the infant cornea is approximately 49.50 to 47 D in the first 1 to 2 months of life in full-term infants, and flattens to normal adult values of 43 to 44 D by 4 years of age.[2]

Lens Diameter and Thickness

The average corneal diameter of an infant to 3 years of age is 10.2 mm. The hydrophilic lens should have a 1 mm limbus-to-lens edge dimension. Therefore, hydrophilic soft lenses should be semi-scleral, using diameters ranging from 12.5 to 13 mm. Gas permeable lenses should fit with a 1 mm corneal limbus-to-lens edge. In most cases, this would be a diameter range of 8.0 to 8.5 mm.

Both the center and edge of the lens must be thick enough and correctly proportioned so that insertion is easy and tearing is minimized. Thin lenses are undesirable for young children because of handling and durability problems.

Aftercare

A child's eyes change dynamically in regards to refractive error, ocular size and shape, and corneal topography. This necessitates more frequent evaluations and contact lens alterations.

Aftercare examinations are determined by a number of factors. These include the child's diagnosis, age of the child, competency of the parents, and progress of the treatment. It is advisable to see the child 24 hours after the lens is dispensed. The patient should be seen again at 1 week, 1 month, and 2 months. Once all is stable, follow-up at 3 month intervals is recommended.

The aftercare examination should include:

1) An assessment of vision in each eye by age-appropriate methods.

2) A re-evaluation of lens fit. Changes can occur rapidly, especially in infants.

3) An assessment of the health of the eye. If possible use a hand-held slit lamp or a loupe and a penlight to inspect the anterior segment. If the child objects to this part of the exam, you must persevere until an accurate assessment is completed.

4) Assess any difficulties the parents and child are having with contact lenses. These include:
  a) Technical problems
      Difficulty in fitting lens
      Lens ejection and loss
      Lens damage
      Corneal insult
      Changes in refractive error
  b) Non-technical problems
      Difficulty in patching (in cases of amblyopia)
      Availability and cost of lenses
      Behavioral problems in the patient
      Family problems
      Developmental problems

Additionally, the parents should be questioned about handling and care of the lenses and the child's response to the treatment. Family support and compliance to instructions is critical.

Adult Aphakic Contact Lens Fitting

In the majority of situations an intraocular lens will be inserted after the removal of the cataract. However, some cases still require an aphakic contact lens fitting (Table 12-2).

Lens selection will not only be premised by the visual needs of the patient but by the patient's physical dexterity and intellectual awareness. If the patient is unable to insert, remove, or care for the lenses, a family member or healthcare aide will need to assist. The individual who assists the patient will need to be taught proper lens maintenance.

Material selection should complement the need for flexible or extended wear use. This would bias lens fitting to hydrophilic over rigid lenses. However, rigid lenses of a high Dk material and thin design would also be acceptable. Any lens design will be a high plus power with an increased mass and anterior surface convexity. These factors can lead to many difficulties and problems as seen in Table 12-3.

Power adjustments should be made based on the over-refraction, using a diagnostic lens with vertex distance compensation. Bitoric designs and/or spectacle overcorrection may be considered for cylindrical requirements. When ordering the final lens, specify a front or back vertex power. If not specified, the final power may vary by approximately 1 to 2 diopters.

Hydrogel Lenses for Adult Aphakia

Fitting hydrophilic lenses for the non-astigmatic aphakic patient is no different than fitting high plus lenses for the phakic patient. The major advantage of using a hydrogel lens is a variable wear schedule and a higher level of comfort, as compared to rigid lenses. Required powers and parameters are available through numerous suppliers. If significant astigmatism is present, the fitter can order customized plus toric lenses.

Hydrophilic lenses are contraindicated when the patient has a history of immunocompromise, corneal vascularization, and/or endothelial compromise.

The initial soft lens of choice has a high water content and an overall lens diameter of approximately 13.8 to 15 mm. The BC should be approximately 1 mm to 1.3 mm flatter than the mean

Table 12-2.
Cases Requiring an Aphakic Contact Lens Fitting

Pediatric aphakia
Intraocular or traumatic disease
Chronic uveitis
Abnormal congenital ocular anatomy
Iris coloboma or aniridia
Ocular trauma
Iridodialysis or iridodonesis
Vascular disease (ie, diabetes)
Surgical complications

Table 12-3.
Difficulties and Complications Associated with Aphakic Contact Lenses

Hypoxia associated with increased lens thickness
Lens loss or lens ejection
Lens dislocation
Decreased vision
Difficult handling
Difficult I & R
Contact lens related infection
Edge fluting
Increased lens awareness

corneal curve. The lens should demonstrate adequate movement in primary, upward, and lateral gazes, as well as complete corneal coverage.

Gas Permeable Contact Lenses for Adult Aphakia

Rigid lens fitting in aphakia does not vary from basic rigid lens techniques other than compensating for the weight associated with a high plus lens. The fitter can choose to design a small and steep lens in order to centralize it, or a larger lens to encourage a lid attachment fit. In either case, the lens design requires a minus lenticular carrier in order to get rid of the sharp edge of the lens and to allow for proper lid interaction.[3,4]

A small lens design is constructed with a steeper BC that allows the lens to center over the visual axis. The problem is that the visual axis may be *decentered* due to surgical reconstruction of the pupil. Any decentration of the lens will lead to poor visual results.

When fitting a small aphakic lens, the mean of the keratometric readings is used to determine the BC. This lens design requires a steeper BC with a larger optic zone. The optic zone should be 0.2 to 0.3 mm larger than the BC, using a bicurve design to limit the lens diameter. The CT needs to be minimized to allow for better centration, but this may increase the potential for peripheral edge dryness. To avoid epithelial drying, a rounded edge with an edge lift of about 11 to 12 mm should be ordered.

Larger lens designs require a lid attachment fit that will enhance comfort and visual stability. The lens should have an overall lens diameter of 8.8 to 9.5 mm with an OZD equal to the BC (or slightly larger by 0.1 to 0.2 mm). The front optic zone should be approximately 2 mm smaller than the overall lens diameter, or about 0.5 mm smaller than the posterior optic zone. The reduction in the OZD will reduce the CT, thereby decreasing the overall weight of the lens. Edge lifts are reduced to approximately 10.5 to 11 mm. The edge lift reduction is compensated for by a minus lenticular carrier to enhance lid attachment.

Larger diameter lenses have the tendency to displace laterally. In this scenario, the overall lens diameter (with the anterior and posterior optic zone) should be increased in equal amounts. This will increase lid grab and reduce lateral displacement. Inferior displacement of a larger lens is due to the added weight. An ultrathin lens with lenticulation can be ordered to reduce the overall weight of the lens.

Patient Instruction

Many of the difficulties with these lenses are due to the patient's inability to see the lens. An ancillary pair of spectacles or a magnification device should be used. I & R problems may require the use of a suction cup or the assistance of another person. Lens loss can also be reduced by instructing the patient to work over a white towel or a mirrored tray. A handling or cosmetic tint is also helpful.

To insert the lens, the patient should bend over, looking down onto the towel or tray, to bring the lens up onto the cornea. (If the patient sits upright and tries to bring the lens onto the eye, the likelihood of dropping the lens increases dramatically.)

If I & R becomes difficult for the patient, the lenses should be prescribed as extended wear and a family member or healthcare assistant will need to help the patient. Otherwise, lens insertion and removal can be done on a regular basis at the clinician's office at 1 or 2 week intervals.

Contact Lenses in Post-Refractive Surgery

A need for postoperative spectacles and/or contact lenses will be required in a substantial percentage of post-refractive surgical patients. Post-refractive surgical fitting of contact lenses is a challenge due to the irregularity of the cornea caused by a flattened corneal cap. Thus, pre and postoperative topographic information and refraction are vitally important.

Before a diagnostic fitting, the patient should be educated regarding potential visual outcomes and expense. The patient who sought out refractive surgery to *avoid* the use of optical appliances may be frustrated by the need for contact lens correction.

For a post-incisional refractive surgical case, a rigid gas permeable lens is preferred in order to avoid the potential adverse reactions (such as incisional neovascularization or ulceration) that can occur with the use of hydrogel lenses.[5] Hydrogel lenses may be considered after a sufficient time has been allotted for wound healing, and should only be used to act as a "pressure bandage" when there is a incisional gap.

The most common concept of fitting post-surgically is to select a trial lens with a CPC based on the presurgical topography or keratometry.[6] An "on K" fit would allow for lid attachment, but would also create edge lift, increased inferior pooling, central clearance, and superior bearing.

The best BC selection would be to apply a "split K" philosophy using the preoperative keratometric readings. A "split K" is simply the average of the keratometry reading. For example, a 44/46 @ 90 average would be 45 diopters, or a 7.5 mm BC. An averaged BC should give mid-peripheral touch with central vaulting (Figure 12-1). Mid-peripheral touch is necessary to support the lens on the least altered mid-peripheral corneal tissue.[7]

Conservatively, the optic zone should be twice as large as the surgical optical zone. The overall lens diameter should allow for lid interaction without creating excessive superior bearing or

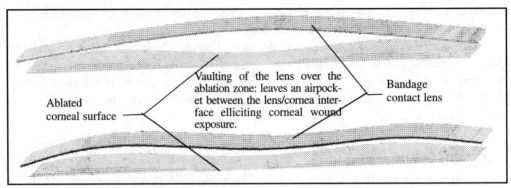

Vaulting of the lens over the ablation zone: leaves an airpocket between the lens/cornea interface elliciting corneal wound exposure.

Bandage contact lens

Ablated corneal surface

Figure 12-1. Alignment and vaulting patterns of bandage contact lenses after photoabulation of the cornea.

inferior lift (ie, 9.2 to 10 mm). PCRs should be employed to allow for the back surface of the lens to contour the anterior peripheral cornea.

If the lens decenters superiorly, either steepen the BC slightly or increase the OZD or the lens diameter. If the diameters are adjusted, 0.2 mm steps are recommended. An alternative is to add base-down prism. If prism is added, 0.75 to 1.25 prism diopters should be used as the initial trial, increasing by 0.5 prism diopter steps as needed, bearing in mind that truncation is not necessary.

If the lens decenters inferiorly, it is necessary to increase lid interaction by increasing the lens diameter and flattening the BC appropriately. Conversely, the lens diameter and CT may be decreased to reduce the weight of the lens and allow it to position more superiorly. Otherwise, a myoflange design will increase the peripheral bulk of the lens and encourage lid grab.

The flattened corneal cap will have a biconvex lens effect, yielding a minus over-refraction. Power adjustments must be made in regards to postsurgical manifest refraction and trial lens over-refraction. Therefore, the trial lens power may mimic the spherical equivalent of the postoperative manifest. Power adjustments should be made without adjusting the lens curvatures or diameters. However, if the BC is adjusted, then a compensation in power is required.[6]

A second method of fitting post-refractive surgery patients is to utilize the philosophy of orthokeratology (or "reverse geometry") and select a flatter lens to enhance the flattened effect of the surgery (if the patient is under-corrected).[8] A flatter BC would be used, with steeper PCRs. If this design is fit, there should be mid-central bearing internal to the mid-periphery. In the case of undercorrection, one can feel comfortable in following an "on K" design with larger optic zone and overall lens diameter.

Another method incorporates the use of mid-peripheral corneal radii at approximately 3.5 mm in the superior periphery.[9] By fitting to a point in the superior periphery, the lens will align in the superior portion of the cornea, allowing the lens to be supported by the upper lid. The lens will decenter superiorly by approximately 1 to 2 mm. After the blink, the lens will be dislodged from the lid and move centrally. The lens will exhibit central fluorescein pooling adjacent to the central clear zone and alignment to the periphery.

The final method of contact lens fitting in such cases is to utilize computerized topographic systems. Once the image has been processed, the operator can select a contact lens design option from the main menu. The program will list corneal statistics. In addition, the fitter can design the lens on the computer utilizing all the necessary parameters and even a simulated fluorescein pattern.

Therapeutic Bandage Contact Lenses

Hydrophilic contact lenses have been used for many years as bandages for various corneal disorders (Tables 12-4, 12-5, 12-6, and 12-7). These disorders include basement membrane dystrophies, recurrent erosion, and chemical burns, as well as postoperative management of photorefractive procedures. The hydrogel bandage lens provides an increase in surface wetting, fosters a more regular refracting surface for superficial corneal irregularities, reduces exposure sensitivity, assists in wound healing, and splints corneal defects such as abrasions or perforations.

High water content and/or ultrathin extended wear materials are generally used. (High water content lenses are traditionally used for non-traumatic disorders. Medium to low water content lenses are used to splint or support a compromised cornea.)

Disposable contact lenses have become popular as bandage lenses due to their convenience, packaging, and cost efficiency. However, they do not have FDA indications for uses other than refractive vision correction in either daily or extended wear.

The optimal lens of choice for a therapeutic use is one with a moderate to high water content, a moderate amount of "stiffness," and as thin as possible. If the lens is too thick, significant corneal edema may be induced. A thin lens may flex or vault off the cornea surface, inducing additional trauma and dehydration. If a lens demonstrates excessive movement, it will chafe and prolong wound healing. In order to prevent lens dehydration, hypotonic preparations should be avoided when wearing a bandage lens.

Lens selection for wound healing assistance is based on the severity and etiology of the corneal disorder, the level of pain, and visual requirements. It is essential to consider oxygen permeability and thickness. If a lens is of low water content it must be an ultrathin design (versus a high water content, which would be slightly thicker).

Hydrogel lenses can also be used as a vehicle for drug delivery. Topical solutions can be substituted for saline as a soak in a contact lens storage container. This saturates the contact lens with the medicinal solution.[10]

Keratoconus

Keratoconus is a non-inflammatory, bilateral, progressive thinning of the cornea leading to an apical protrusion, subsequent scarring, and distorted and decreased vision. Pathological keratoconus involves a breakdown in the integrity of Bowman's membrane with a subsequent loss of stromal substance, leading to anterior stromal scarring and vision loss. If tissue compromise progresses, tears in Descemet's membrane can occur, leading to an influx of aqueous (hydrops).

Contact lenses for keratoconus should contour the corneal shape, yielding a balance of bearing and clearance across the corneal surface (Table 12-8). Contact lenses act as both optical correction and therapeutic aid. The lens must exert a sufficient amount of pressure on the apex to reshape the deformed cornea. However, the fitter should always remember that there is a fine balance between visual improvement and comfort, as well as avoiding contact lens-induced keratitis or scarring.

Piggyback Lens Correction for Keratoconus

Soft lens correction of keratoconus is limited to early onset disease because soft lenses (in general) are not able to exert the appropriate pressure on the corneal surface required to retard the

Table 12-4.

Indications for Therapeutic Bandage Contact Lenses

General Purpose	Specific Indication
Mechanical/structural	Protective barrier, pressure/sealant, structural reinforcement, corneal shape alteration, cicatrix prevention
Symptom relief	Pain control, visual function
Assistance in wound healing	Inhibition of chemotaxis, promotion of re-epithelialization, prevention of epithelial dryness
Drug delivery system	Antibiotic delivery

Adapted from McDermott ML, et al. Therapeutic uses of contact lenses. Surv Ophthalmol. *March/April 1989;33(5):385.*

Table 12-5.

Conditions Warranting Therapeutic Bandage Contact Lenses

Long-term treatment (> 12 months)	Chemical burns, trichiasis, bullous keratopathy, mucous membrane pathology (ie, erythema multiforme)
Medium wear (2 to 12 months)	Bullous keratopathy, corneal exposure, corneal thinning
Short-term (< 2 months)	Vernal keratoconjunctivitis, wound leakage, entropion, delayed corneal re-epithelialization
Recurrent wear	Recurrent erosion, Thygeson's, superficial punctate keratopathy

Adapted from Jackson JA, et al. Therapeutic contact lenses and their use in the management of anterior segment pathology. Journal of the British Contact Lens Association. *1996;19(1):11-19.*

Table 12-6.

Indications and Uses for Therapeutic Bandage Contact Lenses

Condition	Use of Therapeutic Contact Lenses
Acute glaucoma	Delivery of therapeutic agents (ie, pilocarpine, timolol)
Amblyopia	Occlusion therapy
Aniridia	Occlusion/UV protection
Nystagmus	Improvement and stability of visual acuity
Diplopia	Occlusion therapy
Keratopathy (ie, bullous, recurrent erosion, filamentary, Thygeson's, SLK)	Delivery of therapeutic agents and protective patching
Abrasions	Splint and delivery of therapeutic agents
Aphakia	Vision correction and postoperative delivery of therapeutic and analgesic agents
Corneal dystrophy (ie, Fuch's, iridocorneal, posterior polymorphous)	Pain control via protective patching
Chemical injuries (ie, alkali—acid burns)	Delivery of therapeutic agents, protective patching, retardation of toxic and proteolytic cellular processes.
UV and/or post radiation keratopathy (ie, solar, x-rays, PUVA therapy)	Delivery of therapeutic agents, protective patching, and analgesic control
Lid defects (ie, coloboma, trichiasis)	Corneal protection

Table 12-6 continued.

Facial nerve palsy, lagophthalmos	Protection against exposure
Glaucoma—filtering (bleb) procedures	Pressure support on leaking bleb
Keratoplastic management	Protection of graft (cheesewiring—erosion of sutures through graft) Enhancement of graft epithelialization Wound dehiscence (prevention of leakage)
Ulceration (ie, Mooren's)	Delivery of therapeutic agents, protective patching, and analgesic control
Neuroparalytic keratitis (trigeminal anesthesia)	Control of punctate keratopathy (stage one)
Corneal perforation (ie, trauma, stromal lysis, supporative keratopathy)	Delivery of therapeutic agents, protective patching, and analgesic control
Retinal disease (ie, RP*, ROP*)	Low vision assistance, improvement in visual acuity

RP = retinitis pigmentosa, ROP = retinopathy of prematurity

Table 12-7.
FDA Approved Therapeutic Bandage Contact Lenses

Lens Name	Material/Water Content
Soflens (B&L)	Polymacon/38%
Softcon EW or Protek (CIBA)	Vifilcon A/55%
Permalens (Coopervision)	Perfilcon A/70%
Hydrocurve II (PBH—Wesley Jessen)	Bufilcon A/55%
CSI—FW (PBH—Wesley Jessen)	Crofilcon A/38.5%

Table 12-8.
Fitting Options for Keratoconus

- Spectacles
- Soft contact lenses
- Rigid gas permeable or hard contact lenses
- Piggy back designs
- Scleral lenses
- Penetrating keratoplasty

Figure 12-2. Piggyback system for keratoconus.

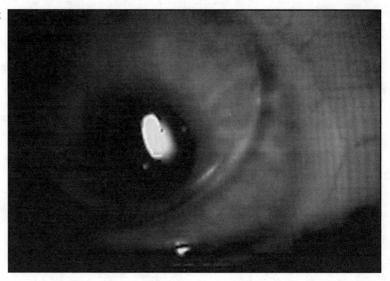

progression of the disease. A soft lens may be a good option, however, when initially introducing a keratoconus patient to contact lens wear.

Soft lenses are best utilized as a carrier for a rigid or hard lens (known as a "piggyback system"). A piggyback system uses an ultrathin hydrogel lens as a supportive carrier. A rigid lens is then worn on top of the hydrogel lens (Figure 12-2).

Using a soft lens as the carrier provides a protective barrier that enhances the patient's comfort. Optically, the soft and rigid contact lens combination increases the usable central optical region of the cornea. Improvement in vision comes from the bearing of the rigid lens on the cornea while being supported by the soft lens. The bracing effect of the rigid lens also prevents and retards the progression of the cone formation.

The fitting of a piggyback soft/rigid lens system should not be any more complicated than the standard rigid lens fitting for keratoconus (discussed next). The only difference in the piggyback system is the presence of the hydrogel lens. The hydrogel lens reduces the difference (minimally to moderately) between the central and peripheral corneal curvatures. This relationship allows the fitter to use a slightly flatter BC for the rigid lens than could be used with the rigid lens alone.

Select a hydrogel lens that covers the cornea completely. The lens diameter should be 1.0 to 1.5 mm from the limbus to lens edge without fluting. Second, the hydrogel lens should demonstrate adequate (but not excessive) movement in primary gaze. (An excessively steep lens will bind to the eye and lead to hydrogel-related corneal complications and hypoxia.)

The rigid contact lens selected for the piggyback system should be fit *approximately equal to or slightly flatter than the average keratometric value prior to hydrogel lens insertion.* An averaged keratometric value can also be obtained *over* the hydrogel lens to determine the BC of the rigid lens. The rigid lens is allowed to demonstrate a greater amount of central bearing as compared to a standard keratoconic design due to the protection of the hydrogel lens. The rigid lens should be designed with minimal CT and ET in order to avoid physiological compromise and to assist in its centration.[11]

To evaluate a piggyback system, a macromolecular fluorescein such as Fluoresoft (Wesley-Jessen, Des Plaines, IL) is recommended. The fluorescein pattern of an acceptable fit should demonstrate minimal to mild central bearing with mid-peripheral clearance and minimal peripheral bearing. The presence of air bubbles underneath the rigid lens indicates that the lens is steep, while bubbles within the PCR and edge indicates an excessively flat fit. The rigid lens will bind to the soft lens, reducing excessive movement and lens awareness. However, the rigid lens will still seek a position over the steeper conical region, exhibited as an inferior displacement.

Another option in the piggyback system is the countersunk or duo-lens system. In this design the hydrogel lens is a 14.5 to 15 mm hydrogel carrier lens with a groove in the central portion. A rigid lens is placed within the countersink groove. The rigid gas permeable lens thickness and the tear reservoir should be equal to the depth of the groove. (Dislocation of the lens is usually due to excessive thickness where the lens protrudes from the groove.) The rigid lens is generally 0.1 to 0.2 mm smaller than the groove's diameter.

An alternative to a piggyback system is a hybrid design. The hybrid design, marketed as a Softperm (Wesley-Jessen, Des Plaines, IL) utilizes a rigid lens fused to a 25% HEMA (hydroxyethylmethacrylate) hydrophilic. The soft HEMA skirt supports the rigid lens, levering the rigid lens away from the corneal surface. Softperm lenses are fit steeper than "flat K." This creates a lacrimal lens that will correct most of any corneal cylinder present.

Adjustments are made to assure proper movement (approximately 0.2 to 0.3 mm) in primary gaze. The BC relationship should be steep enough to allow for complete alignment to mild vaulting over the cornea, yet not so steep that the lens will bind. If the lens is flat, the HEMA skirt will slightly evert and force the rigid lens to bind to the cornea. Uncorrected cylinder can be reduced by a steeper BC. Residual lenticular cylinder will not be corrected and requires a spectacle overcorrection.[12]

Gas Permeable Lens Designs for Keratoconus

There are basically three fitting philosophies for rigid gas permeable lens wear in keratoconus. These are apical bearing, three-point touch, and apical clearance. Apical bearing allows the lens to exert pressure on the cornea surface and flatten the apical region (the usable optical area). Three-point touch allows enough apical touch (or bearing) to enhance vision while leaving a fine balance of clearance to avoid long-term complications. Apical clearance vaults the cone. It is a small lens design that decreases lens awareness while encouraging centration of the lens over the displaced apical region.

Apical Bearing

Apical bearing is a quick fix for vision but inappropriate for long-term comfort. It is associated with frequent lens loss, persistent keratitis, lens awareness, and possible scarring. This lens design exerts pressure on the surface of the cornea while flattening the apical region, thereby reducing a majority of irregular astigmatism and increasing the usable optical area of the cornea. The lens has a relatively large lens diameter that enhances lid attachment but may cause an inferior lens lift. The PCR system is generally 1 to 2 mm flatter than standard PCRs. This fitting method is generally inappropriate, but is often used by the inexperienced keratoconic lens fitter due to the optimal visual results.

Apical Clearance

Apical clearance is a method that requires a design that will vault and clear the apical cornea. The initial BC is selected to equal the steep keratometric value. The lens is designed with a small optic zone, usually equal to or smaller than the BC, with a uniquely small overall lens diameter (sometimes referred to as a "mini-lente" design). This design enhances comfort while encouraging centration over the displaced apical region. This method works best with centralized nipple cones that have a smaller, limited area of irregularity.

The major drawback of this design is less-than-optimal visual acuity as compared to apical bearing. However, the improved comfort and decreased incidence of complications afforded by this design are a tremendous benefit. When using an apical clearance design, an ancillary pair of spectacles may be needed to assist in undercorrected vision.

Three-Point Touch

The three-point touch method is the ultimate compromise of apical clearance and apical touch. It takes into account that a sufficient amount of apical touch or bearing is required to enhance vision, while a fine balance of clearance is needed to avoid long-term complications and to enhance the patient's comfort. Three-point touch is best utilized when there is a centralized or nipple cone, or a slightly inferior displaced cone.

Three-point touch implies that the lens is supported on the cornea via a central bearing, plus two additional points of touch in the periphery along the horizontal meridian.[13] The design of the lens allows for subtle apical touch, mild to moderate paracentral clearance, extra-peripheral touch, and mild peripheral clearance. This distributes the weight of the lens while decreasing "lens rocking."

When designing a three-point touch, care should be taken to avoid a large area of either bearing or clearance. Excessive bearing will enhance vision but decrease comfort and induce punctate staining. Excessive clearance will allow comfort but decrease vision and may induce a "seal" around the cone, leaving an impression ring as well as causing decreased fluid exchange.

The lens design requires a small optic zone equal to or slightly greater than the final BC. The BC is selected to allow centralized alignment to bearing on the 2 to 3 mm central apex. Based on the desired overall lens diameter and lid relationship, two to four PCRs will be incorporated, which are flattened in approximately 0.8 to 1 mm steps. This design allows for a proper tear exchange and prevents seal-off or lens adhesion.

Aspheric Lenses

Aspheric lenses flatten gradually based on an E value that is approximately 0.65 for the normal cornea. A decrease in the E value will maintain a steeper contour, complementing the conical surface. The aspheric design assists in aligning the lens over the cone, thus stabilizing vision.

The fluorescein pattern should exhibit a subtle alignment to bearing, while the peripheral region should show clearance. The major advantage of an aspheric design is to minimize para-apical or peripheral bearing. Several aspheric lenses are available: Envision (Bausch & Lomb, Claremont, Calif), Conforma (Ellip-See-Con), and the VFL II and KAS (GBF Contact Lens, Inc.).

Specialized Designs for Keratoconus

There are several specialized fitting systems for keratoconus including the Soper Lens System, Maguire, Nicone, and Rose K. Each utilizes multiple spherical curve systems that contour the corneal surface. The central apical curve is generally steep, aligning itself with the cone. The mid-periphery and PCRs incorporate a mild to abruptly flatter system to complement the topography of the cornea.

The Soper lens system is bicurve (BC and PCR), where the fitting is based on sagittal depth. The concept is to capture the conical region within the optic zone. The basic diagnostic lens design is based on the severity of the cone; the more advanced the cone, the larger the diameter and the steeper the BC. Mild cones are fit with a lens diameter of 7.4 mm with a 6.0 mm optic zone, moderate cones are fit with 8.5 mm lens diameter with a 7.0 optic zone, and severe or advanced cones are fit with a 9.5 lens diameter with an 8.0 mm optic zone.

The major disadvantage of this system is that the PCR remains constant (7.5 mm) for all lenses regardless of the BC's steepness. This can cause lens binding, fluid stasis, difficult removal, and ring impressions.

The Maguire system utilizes four PCRs. This allows for peripheral clearance that increases fluid exchange, decreases the potential for lens binding, and reduces the incidence of impression rings.[14] This system is fit with slightly smaller diameters and optic zones than the Soper lens. A centralized nipple cone is fit with a 8.1 mm diameter and a 5.5 mm optic zone. A larger, oval cone is fit with a 8.6 mm diameter and a 6 mm optic zone. Finally, a globus cone is fit with a 9.1 mm diameter and 6.5 mm optic zone.

The Nicone System has three BCs and a single PCR system of 12.25 mm. Each BC is unique to that portion of the cornea, determined by a specific formulation.

The primary BC is formulated to conform to the apical region of the cone (K values of 40 to 52 D). The second BC is formulated to prevent traumatization of the ectatic tissue (K values of 53 to 65 D). The third is designed to complement the peripheral cornea (65 D or greater). This curve set-up improves visual acuity and comfort. However, these lenses are difficult to fit due to patented design issues and the inability to specify the needed curvatures for modification of the fit.

The Rose K is the newcomer to specialized designs. This design is based on the identification of disease progression as related to the continual shrinking of the optic zone. The lens design is based on a mathematical model that can generate a multitude of PCRs. These curves will be dependent on the BC, desired edge lift, power, and overall diameter. The Rose K lens system utilizes a 26-lens fitting set.

The lens is fit approximately 0.2 mm steeper than the average keratometric value. It is important to optimize the BC and central fit prior to fitting the periphery. The peripheral system of the lens is based on the desired edge lift. If the edge lift is insufficient, order an increased lift for the final lens. The central fluorescein should exhibit a "feather touch."

References

1. Cutler SI, Nelson LB, Calhoun JH. Extended wear contact lenses in pediatric aphakia. *J Pediatr Ophthalmol Strabismus.* May/June 1985;22:86.

2. Rogers GL. Extended wear silicone contact lenses in children with cataracts. *Ophthalmology.* 1980;87:867.

3. Davis LJ. Contact lens correction of aphakia. In: Bennett E, ed. *Clinical Contact Lens Practice.* Philadelphia, Pa: Lippincott & Co; 1995.

4. Mackie IA. *Medical Contact Practice: A Systematic Approach.* Boston, Mass: Butterworth-Heinemann; 1993.

5. Shivitz IA. Fitting contact lenses after radial keratotomy. *Contact Lens Forum.* December 1988;13:38-39.

6. Shivitz IA, Arrowsmith PN, Russell BM. Contact lenses in the treatment of patients with overcorrected radial keratotomy. *Ophthalmology.* August 1987;94(8):899-903.

7. Seigel IM. Post RK contact lens fitting. *Contact Lens Spectrum.* April 1992;7:41-45.

8. Aquavella JV, Shovlin JP, DePaolis MD. Contact lenses and refractive surgery. In: Harris MG, ed. *Problems of Optometry.* December 1990;2(4):685-693.

9. McDonnell PJ. Computerized analysis of the corneal topography as an aid in fitting contact lenses after radial keratotomy. *Ophthalmic Surg.* January 1992;23(1):55-59.

10. McDermott ML, Chandler JW. Therapeutic uses of contact lenses. *Surv Ophthalmol.* March/April 1989;33(5):381-394.

11. Soper JW. Fitting keratoconus with piggyback and Saturn II lenses. *Contact Lens Forum.* August 1986;11:25-30.

12. Daniels KM, Mariscotti C, McLin A. Independent clinical evaluation of the Softperm lens. *Contact Lens Spectrum.* March 1991;6:41-49.

13. Bennett ES. A common sense approach to fitting keratoconus with RGP lenses. *Optometry Today.* March 1997;5:25-27.

14. Caroline PJ, Doughman DJ, McGuire JR. A new contact lens design for keratoconus: a continuing report. *Contact Lens Journal.* 1978;12:17-20.

Appendix

Abbreviations

AOZ	anterior optical zone		JND	just noticable difference
AOZD	anterior optic zone diameter			
ARE	acute red eye		K	keratometric value
BC	base curve		L	center thickness
BD	base down (prism)		LARS	left add right subtract
BSD	back surface debris			
			MA	manifest astigmatism
CAC	central anterior curve			
CACT	computer assisted corneal topography		NaCl	sodium chloride
			NaFl	sodium fluorescein
CPC	central posterior curve			
CT	center thickness		OSHA	Occupational Safety and Health Administration
D	diameter		OZD	optic zone diameter
D	diopters		OZR	optic zone radius
DC	diopters of cylinder			
Deq	spherical equivalent		PCR	posterior curve
Dk	oxygen permeability		pH	the acidic or basic property of a material
Dk/L	oxygen transmissibility			
DS	diopters of sphere		PMMA	polymethylmethacrylate
			POZD	posterior optic zone diameter
e value	eccentricity			
EDTA	ethylene diamine tetra-acetic acid		rpm	revolutions per minute
EOP	equivalent oxygen percent			
ET	edge thickness		SA	silicone acrylate
			SAM	steeper add minus
FAP	flatter add plus		SCO	spherocylindrical over-refraction
FDA	Food and Drug Administration		SCR	secondary curve
FSA	fluorinated silicone acrylate		SEI	subepithelial infiltrates
			SLK	superior limbic keratitis
GP	gas permeable		SPK	superficial punctate keratitis
GPC	giant papillary conjunctivitis		ST	straight top
HEMA	hydroxyethylmethacrylate		UV	ultraviolet
HIV	human immunodeficiency virus			
			VLK	vascularized limbic keratitis
I & R	insertion and removal			
ICR	intermediate curve			
IRA	internal residual astigmatism			

Table A-1.

Keratometer Extension Chart

Steep Curve (+1.25 D lens over aperture)				Flat Curve (-1.00 D lens over aperture)			
Drum Measurement (D)	True Curve (D)	Drum Measurement (D)	True Curve (D)	Drum Measurement (D)	True Curve (D)	Drum Measurement (D)	True Curve (D)
52.00	61.00	46.87	55.87	42.00	36.00	36.87	30.87
51.87	60.87	46.75	55.75	41.87	35.87	36.75	30.75
51.75	60.75	46.62	55.62	41.75	35.75	36.62	30.62
51.62	60.62	46.50	55.50	41.62	35.62	36.50	30.50
51.50	60.50	46.37	55.37	41.50	35.50	36.37	30.37
51.37	60.37	46.25	55.25	41.37	35.37	36.25	30.25
51.25	60.25	46.12	55.12	41.25	35.25	36.12	30.12
51.12	60.12	46.00	55.00	41.12	35.12	36.00	30.00
51.00	60.00			41.00	35.00		
50.87	59.87	45.87	54.87	40.87	34.87		
50.75	59.75	45.75	54.75	40.75	34.75		
50.62	59.62	45.62	54.62	40.62	34.62		
50.50	59.50	45.50	54.50	40.50	34.50		
50.37	59.37	45.37	54.37	40.37	34.37		
50.25	59.25	45.25	54.25	40.25	34.25		
50.12	59.12	45.12	54.12	40.12	34.12		
50.00	59.00	45.00	54.00	40.00	34.00		
49.87	58.87	44.87	53.87	39.87	33.87		
49.75	58.75	44.75	53.75	39.75	33.75		
49.62	58.62	44.62	53.62	39.62	33.62		
49.50	58.50	44.50	53.50	39.50	33.50		
49.37	58.37	44.37	53.37	39.37	33.37		
49.25	58.25	44.25	53.25	39.25	33.25		
49.12	58.12	44.12	53.12	39.12	33.12		
49.00	58.00	44.00	53.00	39.00	33.00		
48.75	57.75	43.87	52.87	38.87	32.87		
48.62	57.62	43.75	52.75	38.75	32.75		
48.50	57.50	43.62	52.62	38.62	32.62		
48.37	57.37	43.50	52.50	38.50	32.50		
48.25	57.25	43.37	52.37	38.37	32.37		
48.12	57.12	43.25	52.25	38.25	32.25		
48.00	57.00	43.12	52.12	38.12	32.12		
47.87	56.87	43.00	52.00	38.00	32.00		
47.75	56.75			37.87	31.87		
47.62	56.62			37.75	31.75		
47.50	56.50			37.62	31.62		
47.37	58.37			37.50	31.50		
47.25	56.25			37.37	31.37		
47.12	56.12			37.25	31.25		
47.00	56.00			37.12	31.12		
				37.00	31.00		

Table A-2a.
Vertex Distance Chart

Minus Lenses

Spectacle Lens Power	Vertex Distance							
	8.00	9.00	10.00	11.00	12.00	13.00	14.00	15.00
4.00	3.87	3.87	3.87	3.87	3.87	3.75	3.75	3.75
4.50	4.37	4.37	4.25	4.25	4.25	4.25	4.25	4.25
5.00	4.75	4.75	4.75	4.75	4.75	4.75	4.62	4.62
5.50	5.25	5.25	5.25	5.12	5.12	5.12	5.12	5.12
6.00	5.75	5.75	5.62	5.62	5.62	5.62	5.50	5.50
6.50	6.12	6.12	6.12	6.12	6.00	6.00	6.00	5.87
7.00	6.62	6.62	6.50	6.50	6.50	6.37	6.37	6.37
7.50	7.12	7.00	7.00	6.87	6.87	6.87	6.75	6.75
8.00	7.50	7.50	7.37	7.37	7.25	7.25	7.25	7.12
8.59	8.00	7.87	7.87	7.75	7.75	7.62	7.62	7.50
9.00	8.37	8.37	8.25	8.25	8.12	8.00	8.00	7.87
9.50	8.87	8.75	8.62	8.62	8.50	8.50	8.37	8.37
10.00	9.25	9.12	9.12	9.12	9.00	8.87	8.87	8.75
10.50	9.62	9.62	9.50	9.37	9.37	9.25	9.12	9.12
11.00	10.12	10.00	9.87	9.87	9.75	9.62	9.50	9.50
11.50	10.50	10.37	10.37	10.25	10.12	10.00	9.87	9.75
12.00	11.00	10.87	10.75	10.62	10.50	10.37	10.25	10.12
12.50	11.37	11.25	11.12	11.00	10.87	10.75	10.62	10.50
13.00	11.75	11.62	11.50	11.37	11.25	11.12	11.00	10.87
13.50	12.12	12.00	11.87	11.75	11.62	11.50	11.37	11.25
14.00	12.62	12.37	12.25	12.12	12.00	11.87	11.75	11.62
14.50	13.00	12.87	12.62	12.50	12.37	12.25	12.00	11.87
15.00	13.37	13.25	13.00	12.87	12.75	12.50	12.37	12.25
15.50	13.75	13.62	13.37	13.25	13.12	12.87	12.75	12.62
16.00	14.12	14.00	13.75	13.62	13.37	13.25	13.12	12.87
16.50	14.62	14.37	14.12	14.00	13.75	13.62	13.37	13.25
17.00	15.00	14.75	14.50	14.37	14.12	13.87	13.75	13.50
17.50	15.37	15.12	14.87	14.62	14.50	14.25	14.00	13.87
18.00	15.75	15.50	15.25	15.00	14.75	14.62	14.37	14.12
18.50	16.12	15.87	15.62	15.37	15.12	14.87	14.75	14.50
19.00	16.50	16.25	16.00	15.75	15.50	15.25	15.00	14.75

Table A-2b. Vertex Distance Chart

Plus Lenses

Spectacle Lens Power	Vertex Distance							
	8.00	9.00	10.00	11.00	12.00	13.00	14.00	15.00
4.00	4.12	4.12	4.12	4.12	4.25	4.25	4.25	4.25
4.50	4.62	4.75	4.75	4.75	4.75	4.75	4.75	4.87
5.00	5.25	5.25	5.25	5.25	5.37	5.37	5.37	5.37
5.50	5.75	5.75	5.87	5.87	5.87	5.87	6.00	6.00
6.00	6.25	6.37	6.37	6.37	6.50	6.50	6.50	6.62
6.50	6.87	6.87	7.00	7.00	7.00	7.12	7.12	7.25
7.00	7.37	7.50	7.50	7.62	7.62	7.75	7.75	7.87
7.50	8.00	8.00	8.12	8.12	8.25	8.25	8.37	8.50
8.00	8.50	8.62	8.75	8.75	8.87	8.87	9.00	9.12
8.50	9.12	9.25	9.25	9.37	9.50	9.50	9.62	9.75
9.00	9.75	9.75	9.87	10.00	10.12	10.25	10.25	10.37
9.50	10.25	10.37	10.50	10.62	10.75	10.87	11.00	11.12
10.00	10.87	11.00	11.12	11.25	11.37	11.50	11.62	11.75
10.50	11.50	11.62	11.75	11.87	12.00	12.12	12.25	12.50
11.00	12.00	12.25	12.37	12.50	12.62	12.87	13.00	13.12
11.50	12.62	12.87	13.00	13.12	13.37	13.50	13.75	13.87
12.00	13.25	13.50	13.62	13.87	14.00	14.25	14.37	14.62
12.50	13.87	14.12	14.25	14.50	14.75	14.87	15.12	15.37
13.00	14.50	14.75	15.00	15.12	15.37	15.62	15.87	16.12
13.50	15.12	15.37	15.62	15.87	16.12	16.37	16.62	16.87
14.00	15.75	16.00	16.25	16.50	16.87	17.12	17.37	17.75
14.50	16.37	16.62	17.00	17.25	17.50	17.87	18.25	18.50
15.00	17.00	17.37	17.62	18.00	18.25	18.62	19.00	19.37
15.50	17.75	18.00	18.37	18.62	19.00	19.37	19.75	20.25
16.00	18.37	18.75	19.00	19.37	19.75	20.25	20.62	21.00
16.50	19.00	19.37	19.75	20.12	20.62	21.00	21.50	21.87
17.00	19.62	20.12	20.50	20.87	21.37	21.87	22.25	22.87
17.50	20.37	20.75	21.25	21.62	22.12	22.62	23.12	23.75
18.00	21.00	21.50	22.00	22.50	23.00	23.50	24.12	24.62
18.50	21.75	22.25	22.75	23.25	23.75	24.37	25.00	25.62
19.00	22.37	22.87	23.50	24.00	24.62	25.25	25.87	26.62

Table A-3.
Conversion of Diopters to Millimeters of Radius

Diopters	mm	Diopters	mm	Diopters	mm	Diopters	mm
20.00	16.875	39.00	8.653	45.00	7.500	51.00	6.617
22.00	15.340	39.12	8.627	45.12	7.480	51.12	6.602
24.00	14.062	39.25	8.598	45.25	7.458	51.25	6.585
26.00	12.980	39.37	8.572	45.37	7.438	51.37	6.569
27.00	12.500	39.50	8.544	45.50	7.417	51.50	6.553
28.00	12.053	39.62	8.518	45.62	7.398	51.62	6.538
29.00	11.638	39.75	8.490	45.75	7.377	51.75	6.521
29.50	11.441	39.87	8.465	45.87	7.357	51.87	6.506
30.00	11.250	40.00	8.437	46.00	7.336	52.00	6.490
30.50	11.065	40.12	8.412	46.12	7.317	52.12	6.475
31.00	10.887	40.25	8.385	46.25	7.297	52.25	6.459
31.50	10.714	40.37	8.360	46.37	7.278	52.37	6.444
32.00	10.547	40.50	8.333	46.50	7.258	52.50	6.428
32.50	10.385	40.62	8.308	46.62	7.239	52.62	6.413
33.00	10.227	40.75	8.282	46.75	7.219	52.75	6.398
33.50	10.075	40.87	8.257	46.87	7.200	52.87	6.383
34.00	9.926	41.00	8.231	47.00	7.180	53.00	6.367
34.25	9.854	41.12	8.207	47.12	7.162	53.12	6.353
34.50	9.783	41.25	8.181	47.25	7.142	53.25	6.338
34.75	9.712	41.37	8.158	47.37	7.124	53.37	6.323
35.00	9.643	41.50	8.132	47.50	7.105	53.50	6.308
35.25	9.574	41.62	8.109	47.62	7.087	53.62	6.294
35.50	9.507	41.75	8.083	47.75	7.068	53.75	6.279
35.75	9.440	41.87	8.060	47.87	7.050	53.87	6.265
36.00	9.375	42.00	8.035	48.00	7.031	54.00	6.250
36.12	9.343	42.12	8.012	48.12	7.013	54.12	6.236
36.25	9.310	42.25	7.998	48.25	6.994	54.25	6.221
36.37	9.279	42.37	7.965	48.37	6.977	54.37	6.207
36.50	9.246	42.50	7.941	48.50	6.958	54.50	6.192
36.62	9.216	42.62	7.918	48.62	6.941	54.62	6.179
36.75	9.183	42.75	7.894	48.75	6.923	54.75	6.164
36.87	9.153	42.87	7.872	48.87	6.906	54.87	6.150
37.00	9.121	43.00	7.878	49.00	6.887	55.00	6.136
37.12	9.092	43.12	7.826	49.12	6.870	55.12	6.123
37.25	9.060	43.25	8.803	49.25	6.852	55.25	6.108
37.37	9.031	43.37	7.781	49.37	6.836	55.37	6.095
37.50	9.000	43.50	7.758	49.50	6.818	55.50	6.081
37.62	8.971	43.62	7.737	49.62	6.801	55.62	6.068
37.75	8.940	43.75	7.714	49.75	6.783	55.75	6.054
37.87	8.912	43.87	7.693	49.87	6.767	55.87	6.041
38.00	8.881	44.00	7.670	50.00	6.750	56.00	6.027
38.12	8.853	44.12	7.649	50.12	6.733	56.50	5.973
38.25	8.823	44.25	7.627	50.25	6.716	57.00	5.921
38.37	8.795	44.37	7.606	50.37	6.700	57.50	5.869
38.50	8.766	44.50	7.584	50.50	6.683	58.00	5.819
38.62	8.738	44.62	7.563	50.62	6.667	58.50	5.769
38.75	8.708	44.75	7.541	50.75	6.650	59.00	5.720
38.87	8.682	44.87	7.521	50.87	6.634	60.00	5.625

Index

Encourage education, refine office knowledge, and increase office efficiency with *The Basic Bookshelf for Eyecare Professionals series*.

The Basic Bookshelf for Eyecare Professionals

Title	Author	Book#	Price
☐ Basic Procedures	DuBois	63470	$30.00
☐ Cataract and Glaucoma	Duvall	63357	$24.00
☐ COA Exam Review Manual	Ledford	63330	$33.00
☐ COMT Exam Review Manual	Ledford	64221	$33.00
☐ COT Exam Review Manual	Ledford	63241	$33.00
☐ Clinical Ocular Photography	Cunningham	63772	$30.00
☐ Contact Lenses	Daniels	63454	$30.00
☐ Emergencies in Eyecare	Hargis	63543	$30.00
☐ Frames and Lenses	Carlton	63640	$30.00
☐ General Medical Knowledge	Bittinger	63349	$30.00
☐ Instrumentation for Eyecare Paraprofessionals	Herrin	63993	$30.00
☐ Low Vision Handbook, The	Brown	63292	$30.00
☐ Ocular Anatomy and Physiology	Lens	63489	$30.00
☐ Office and Career Management	Borover	63314	$30.00
☐ Ophthalmic Medications and Pharmacology	Duvall	63284	$26.00
☐ Ophthalmic Surgical Assistant, The	Boess-Lott	64035	$30.00
☐ Optics, Retinoscopy, and Refractometry	Lens	63977	$30.00
☐ Overview of Ocular Disorders	Gwin	63365	$30.00
☐ Overview of Ocular Surgery and Surgical Counseling	Pickett	63322	$30.00
☐ Quick Reference Glossary, 2E	Hoffman	63705	$22.00
☐ Refractive Surgery for Eyecare Paraprofessionals	Gayton	63373	$21.00
☐ Slit Lamp Primer, The	Ledford	63306	$30.00
☐ Special Skills and Techniques	Van Boemel	63497	$30.00
☐ Systematic Approach to Strabismus, A	Hansen	63268	$27.00
☐ Visual Fields	Choplin	63632	$33.00

Subtotal $_____

NJ residents add 6% sales tax $_____

Handling Charge $__4.50__

Total $_____

ORDER TODAY!

Name: _____

Address: _____

City: _____ State: _____ Zip Code: _____

Phone:_____ Fax: _____

Charge my: ___American Express ___Visa ___Mastercard Account#: _____

Exp. date: _____ Signature: _____

Prices are subject to change. Shipping charges may apply.

Mail order form to:
SLACK Incorporated, Professional Book Division, 6900 Grove Road, Thorofare, NJ 08086-9447
Call: (800) 257-8290, (609) 848-1000, or (856) 848-1000 • Fax: (609) 853-5991 or (856) 853-5991
Send an email to orders@slackinc.com • Visit our World Wide Web site at www.slackinc.com
CODE: 6A416

For your information

This book and many others on numerous different topics are available from SLACK Incorporated. For further information or a copy of our latest catalog, contact us at:

Professional Book Division
SLACK Incorporated
6900 Grove Road
Thorofare, NJ 08086 USA
Telephone: 1-609-848-1000, 1-856-848-1000
1-800-257-8290
Fax: 1-609-853-5991, 1-856-853-5991
E-mail: orders@slackinc.com
WWW: http://www.slackinc.com

We accept most major credit cards and checks or money orders in US dollars drawn on a US bank. Most orders are shipped within 72 hours.

Contact us for information on recent releases, forthcoming titles, and bestsellers. If you have a comment about this title or see a need for a new book, direct your correspondence to the Editorial Director at the above address.

If you are an instructor, we can be reached at the address listed above or on the Internet at educomps@slackinc.com for specific needs.

Thank you for your interest and we hope you found this work beneficial.